咨询说明

水烟抽吸

健康影响、研究需求和监管措施

（原著第 2 版）

WHO 烟草制品管制研究小组

主　译　胡清源

副主译　侯宏卫　陈　欢

科学出版社

北　京

图字：01-2017-4847 号

内 容 简 介

世界卫生组织（WHO）烟草制品管制研究小组（TobReg）关于水烟抽吸的咨询说明出版十年来，越来越多的证据表明，抽吸水烟引发的患病率和不良健康影响持续增长，鉴于此，WHO 无烟草行动组（TFI）发布关于水烟抽吸的咨询说明第 2 版。本咨询说明旨在对抽吸水烟（可追溯到至少 400 年前的非洲和亚洲）引发的患病率增加和潜在健康影响给予更多的关注。本咨询说明是应 2014 年 10 月在俄罗斯莫斯科召开的 WHO《烟草控制框架公约》第六次缔约方会议提请 WHO 的要求而编写，将使 WHO 成员国和研究机构更全面地了解水烟抽吸的健康影响。

本书会引起吸烟与健康、烟草化学和公共卫生学等诸多应用领域的科学家的兴趣，也为客观评价烟草制品的管制和披露提供必要的参考。

图书在版编目(CIP)数据

咨询说明：水烟抽吸：健康影响、研究需求和监管措施：原书第2版/WHO烟草制品管制研究小组编；胡清源主译. —北京：科学出版社, 2018.1

书名原文：Advisory note: Waterpipe tobacco smoking: health effects, research needs and recommended actions for regulators (2nd ed)

ISBN 978-7-03-056058-2

I.①咨⋯ II.①W⋯ ②胡⋯ III.①水烟 – 吸烟 – 影响 – 健康 – 研究 IV.①R163.2

中国版本图书馆CIP数据核字(2017)第314758号

责任编辑：刘 冉 / 责任校对：韩 杨
责任印制：张 伟 / 封面设计：铭轩堂

科 学 出 版 社 出版
北京东黄城根北街 16 号
邮政编码：100717
http://www.sciencep.com

北京教图印刷有限公司 印刷
科学出版社发行 各地新华书店经销
*
2018年1月第 一 版 开本：890 × 1240 A5
2018年1月第一次印刷 印张：4 7/8
字数：150 000
定价：80.00元
（如有印装质量问题，我社负责调换）

Waterpipe tobacco smoking:

health effects, research needs and recommended actions for regulators

2nd edition

WHO Study Group on Tobacco Product Regulation (TobReg)

翻译委员会

主　译： 胡清源

副主译： 侯宏卫　陈　欢

译　者： 胡清源　侯宏卫　陈　欢

　　　　　刘　彤　韩书磊　付亚宁

　　　　　王红娟

目 录

CONTENTS

WHO 烟草制品管制研究小组

成员

D. L. Ashley 博士，美国食品药品管理局（美国马里兰州罗克维尔）烟草制品中心科学办公室主任

O. A. Ayo-Yusuf 教授，Sefako Makgatho 卫生科学大学（南非比勒陀利亚）口腔卫生科学学院院长

A. R. Boobis 教授，英国伦敦帝国学院医学系药理学与治疗学中心生化药理学专业；伦敦帝国学院公共卫生英格兰毒理学课题组组长

Vera Luiza da Costa e Silva 博士，巴西里约热内卢高级公共卫生专家，独立顾问

M. V. Djordjevic 博士，美国国家癌症研究所（美国马里兰州贝塞斯达）癌症控制与人口科学部行为研究处烟草控制研究项目主任／项目负责人

N. Gray 博士，维多利亚癌症委员会（澳大利亚墨尔本）高级荣誉合伙人

P. Gupta 博士， Healis Sekhsaria 公共卫生研究所（印度孟买）所长

S. K. Hammond 博士，加利福尼亚大学伯克利分校（美国加利福尼亚州伯克利）公共卫生学院环境卫生学教授

D. Hatsukami 博士，明尼苏达大学（美国明尼苏达州明尼阿波利斯）精神病学教授

A. Opperhuizen 博士，荷兰乌得勒支省风险评估和研究办公室主任

G. Zaatari 博士，WHO 烟草制品管制研究小组主席；贝鲁特美国大

学（黎巴嫩贝鲁特）病理学与实验医学教授

撰稿人

E. Akl 博士，贝鲁特美国大学（黎巴嫩贝鲁特）内科医学系医学专业副教授

T. Eissenberg 博士，弗吉尼亚联邦大学（美国弗吉尼亚州里士满）烟草制品研究中心心理学教授，联合主任

W. Maziak 博士，佛罗里达国际大学（美国佛罗里达州迈阿密）流行病学系教授，系主任；叙利亚烟草研究中心主任

P. Mehrotra 博士，印度人口委员会（印度新德里）高级项目主管

J. Morton 先生，美国疾病控制与预防中心（美国佐治亚州亚特兰大）吸烟与健康办公室全球烟草控制分部高级调查方法学家

A. Shihadeh 博士，贝鲁特美国大学（黎巴嫩贝鲁特）工程与建筑学院机械工程系教授

WHO 秘书处

（非传染性疾病预防处无烟草行动组，瑞士日内瓦）

M. Aryee-Quansah 女士，行政助理

A. Peruga 博士，计划理事

G. Vestal 女士，技术官员（法律）

1. 前言

烟草制品的管制包括通过测试、规范及强制披露测试结果来监管烟草制品的成分和释放物，以及监管烟草制品的包装和标识，是综合性烟草控制规划的支柱之一。世界卫生组织《烟草控制框架公约》（WHO FCTC）是一项具有约束力的国际条约，在其第 9, 10, 11 条确认了烟草制品管制的重要性，公约缔约方受这些条款的约束。

2000 年，为填补当时的知识空白，世界卫生组织（WHO）成立了一个烟草制品管制科学咨询小组。该小组提供的科学资料成为公约三项条款文本的协商及随后达成共识的基础。

2003 年 11 月，WHO 总干事认识到管制烟草制品的极度重要性，将烟草制品管制特设的科学咨询委员会正式改为一个研究小组，即 WHO 烟草制品管制研究小组（TobReg）。该小组由国家级和国际性的科学专家组成，涉及产品监管、烟草依赖治疗以及烟草组成成分和释放物的实验室分析等领域，其工作是基于烟草制品相关问题的最新研究的科学证据，提出建议及测试，以填补烟草控制方面的监管空白。作为 WHO 的一个正式部门，TobReg 通过总干事向 WHO 执行委员会提交报告，以提请成员国关注 WHO 对烟草制品管制所做出的努力。

应那些有"水烟"这种烟草使用方式的特别接触群体的成员国的要求，TobReg 根据 WHO 无烟草行动组的优先顺序和 WHO FCTC 关于烟草制品管制的规定，发布了咨询说明《水烟抽吸——健康影响、研究需求和监管措施》第 1 版 [1]。2005 年，TobReg 在巴西里约热内卢举行的第二次会议上批准并通过了该咨询说明。自此以后，又获得了新的信息，并着重针对第 1 版存在的不足进行了科学研究。此外，2013 年 10 月在阿布扎比举行的第一届水烟抽吸国际会议讨论了关于这个问题的认识情况；随后，2014 年 10 月在卡塔尔多哈举行了第二次会议，主题是"水烟抽吸研究：水烟和卷烟两种流行趋势的碰撞"。两次会议的与会者呼吁 WHO 更新 2005 年版咨询说明，并考虑采取其他行动支持成员国和 WHO FCTC 缔约方预防和控制水烟的使用及其他形式的烟草暴露。此外，2014 年 3 月，若干 TobReg 成员及地区和国际水烟专家参加了在埃及开罗 WHO 地中海东部地区办事处举行的研讨会，在会上他们讨论了科学证据、挑战、差距和监管政策等议题，并商定撰写咨询说明第 2 版。

WHO 委托致谢中列出的六位撰稿人起草本报告的主干章节。此外，2014 年 10 月，WHO FCTC 缔约方大会在俄罗斯莫斯科举行的第六次会议（COP 6）要求 WHO 编写一份关于水烟烟草制品有害成分和释放物的报告，并提出一份可选用的政策措施及控制水烟烟草制品使用最佳做法的报告，提请 WHO FCTC 第七次缔约方会议（COP 7）审议。因此，WHO 请 TobReg 发布关于水烟抽吸对健康影响、研究需求和监管措施建议的咨询说明第 2 版。第 7 章着重分析水烟有害成分和释放物的健康影响，第 10 章提出政策建议，第 11 章为监管机构提出建议。TobReg 很高兴提交关于水烟抽吸的咨询说明第 2 版。

TobReg 成员以个人身份无偿服务，并不代表政府或其他机构。他们的观点不一定反映 WHO 的决议或声明的政策。这些成员的名字署在本报告中。

2. 致谢

WHO 烟草制品管制研究小组（TobReg）的这份咨询说明的出版要感谢许多人。本咨询说明在 Armando Peruga 博士和 Douglas Bettcher 博士的监督和支持下，由 Gemma Vestal 女士负责协调出版。

特别感谢几位撰稿人，他们与我们一起工作了整整一年，才使得这份咨询说明能够于 2015 年 3 月 17~21 日在阿拉伯联合酋长国阿布扎比举行的第 16 届世界烟草或健康大会水烟第三次全会期间发布。Elie Akl 博士、Thomas Eissenberg 博士、Wasim Maziak 博士、Purnima Mehrotra 博士、Jeremy Morton 博士和 Alan Shihadeh 博士几位撰稿人孜孜不倦地工作，反复修改成稿。

我们对 TobReg 的所有成员表示衷心的感谢，感谢他们全心奉献，始终如一地履行就烟草制品管制这一烟草控制中相当复杂的领域向 WHO 提供建议的承诺。感谢他们花费大量的时间审稿，给予有见地的建议和指导。作为独立专家，TobReg 的成员无偿为 WHO 服务。

感谢 WHO 同事 Miriamjoy Aryee-Quansah 女士、Gareth Burns 先生、Elaine Alexandre Caruana 女士、Luis Madge 先生、Elizabeth Tecson 女士、Rosane Serrao 女士和 Moira Sy 女士在数月的出版周期内提供的行政支持。

特别感谢 WHO 地中海东部地区办公室主任 Ala Alwan 博士及其同事非传染性疾病和心理健康部主任 Samer Jabbour 博士，以及无烟草行动组地区顾问 Fatimah El Awa 博士，他们于 2014 年 3 月 30~31 日在埃及开罗地区办事处召集和主办了本咨询说明第 2 版的筹备研讨会，展现了其远见和领导力。在该次会议上，确定了第 2 版的初始大纲和各章的内容框架。在撰稿人和 TobReg 成员的协作下，针对 WHO FCTC 缔约方大会 2014 年 10 月在俄罗斯莫斯科举行的第六次会议提出的要求，又将内容进行了重新整理。

此外，我们要向 WHO 的编辑、文字编辑和校对员以及葡萄牙的设计和排版人员表达谢意，感谢他们以极大的耐心在紧迫的时间期限内明察秋毫，精益求精。还要感谢美国健康伙伴有限责任公司（Health Partmers, LLC）的 Jon Barnhart 先生创作的封面图片，以及 Christophe Oliver 先生所作中东水烟和"bong"水烟的插图。

最后但同样重要的是，WHO 感谢无烟草行动组的前实习生们为本咨询说明的成果付出了大量的时间，她们是：Aurelie Abrial 女士、Hannah Patzke 女士和 Angeli Vigo 女士。无论她们在未来从事何种光明的事业，我们都希望她们能够在烟草控制的相关方面继续热情工作。

毫无疑问，因为有太多的人参与了本咨询说明工作，有许多人我们在这里没有提及。我们为任何遗漏而深表歉意。我们同时感谢所有署名的和未署名的人。没有你们的帮助和支持，就没有这份咨询说明。非常感谢你们。

3. 目的

　　TobReg 的这份咨询说明旨在对水烟烟草抽吸越来越流行及其潜在的健康影响给予更多关注。本咨询说明的第 1 版在 2005 年出版[1]，已历经了十几年。在此期间，在许多国家和人群中已进行了大量关于水烟健康危害和抽吸日益普遍问题的研究。尽管认识在不断地增加，仍然存在普遍的公众误解，即认为水烟烟草抽吸是某种保护方式或比抽吸卷烟"更安全"。在一些国家，水烟抽吸在某些亚人群中越来越流行，甚至超过了卷烟抽吸。

　　鉴于这种趋势，需要更多的努力，使水烟烟草抽吸政策符合WHO《烟草控制框架公约》要求。本咨询说明的目的是向 WHO 及其成员国提供指导，向监管机构通报实施 WHO《烟草控制框架公约》关于教育和宣传的规定，给出建议性政策并告知消费者水烟抽吸的风险。它还为关注水烟烟草抽吸健康影响的研究人员、研究机构和资助机构提供了更全面的认知。此外，本咨询说明重点关注那些致力于吸烟预防和戒烟的项目，以确保这些项目适应水烟使用的独特性。

4. 背景和历史

　　世界各地有无数种水烟，本咨询说明中涉及的是俗称"水烟筒"（narghileh）、"水烟壶"（shisha）或"水烟袋"（hookah）的水烟，这种水烟在 20 世纪 90 年代全球化。它由水烟头或烟草碗（其中放置烟草）、瓶体、水碗、软管和烟嘴组成（图 1）。水烟头底部的孔使烟雾进入瓶体的中心导管，导管浸没在水（或酒精或软饮料）中，水灌满水碗一半体积。皮革制或塑料软管从水碗的顶部排出，末端是吸嘴，吸烟者从吸嘴吸入烟气。木炭或煤饼[1]被放置在装满烟草的水烟头顶部，通常用打孔的铝箔片与烟草分隔。装上水烟头或烟草碗并点燃木炭后，吸烟者通过软管吸气，将空气吸入木炭及其周围。产生的加热空气也含有木炭的燃烧产物，接着通过烟草，烟草被加热后产生主流烟气气溶胶。烟气穿过水烟瓶体，通过水碗中的水产生气泡，最后通过软管被输送到吸烟者。在抽吸期间，吸烟者通常添加和调节木炭来保持期望的味道和烟气浓度。为此，一堆点燃的木炭可能会保存在附近的火箱中，这可能会导致吸入额外的有害物。吸烟者也可以选择更方便、更易燃的煤块，它可以直接用便携式打火机点燃。因为水烟抽吸的公用性，共享吸嘴，所以还存在传播传染性疾病的可能。

　　1　煤饼有时被用来代替木炭；此后，所有提到的木炭均包括煤饼

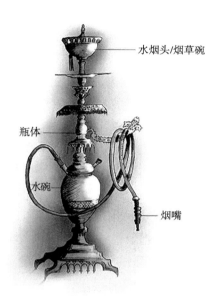

图 1　中东水烟

　　水烟的设计风格存在地区和文化差异，例如水烟头或水碗的尺寸以及吸嘴的个数，但是所有水烟都含有水，烟气在到达吸烟者之前通过这些水。

　　水烟应与被称为"电子水烟袋（e-hookahs）"、"电子水烟壶（e-shisha）"或"水烟笔（hookah pens）"的电子装置区别开来。这些装置属于电子烟碱传输系统，那些加香的产品味道类似于被称为"maassel"的调味烟草。电子装置不使用木炭燃烧；而是用电加热甜味的液体产生可被吸入的气溶胶。目前正在对这些装置进行研究。

　　虽然抽吸卷烟是世界上大多数地区吸烟的主要形式，但水烟使用占全球烟草使用的份额显著地增长。它在亚洲、非洲和中东地区最普遍，在其他大陆也是迅速发展的一个问题。在 WHO 地中海东部地区，水烟的使用在一些国家已经超过了卷烟的使用，男性和女性的使用都越来越多，更严重的是青少年和儿童[2]。

4.1 历　　史

　　水烟被非洲和亚洲土著民用来抽吸烟草和其他物质，如花、香料、水果、咖啡、大麻或大麻提取物，至少有四个世纪了，也许更早[3]。它们的起源有些模糊，但已知是印度和中国的贸易路线促进了在亚洲、中东和非洲部分地区的传播[4]。16 世纪在印度使用的水烟是用椰子壳作为储水容器，顶部插入一个竹苇[4]。这种类型的椰壳水烟被普通人使用，而富裕家庭的吸烟者使用具有华丽设计的黄铜水烟[5]。根据历史记载[6]，水烟是在印度阿克巴大帝统治期间（1556~1605 年）由一名内科医生发明的，据称是为了降低烟草的有害性。这位名叫哈基姆·阿布·法特赫（Hakim Abul Fath）的医生建议烟草的"烟雾应当首先通过一个小型的装水容器从而变得无害。"[5, 6] 因此，"这样做是相对安全的"这个看法可能和水烟本身一样古老，这一广泛流传却未经证实的信念直到今天仍被许多水烟用户所相信[7]。

4.2　近　　况

　　水烟可以从专卖店（包括互联网供应商）购买，专卖店也供应木炭、烟草和配件。有时被销售的水烟是便携式的，配有诸如携带用带或箱的配件。一些声称可降低烟雾危害的配件也在销售，例如含有活性炭或棉的吸嘴、可加入到水碗中的化学添加剂以及可产生较小气泡的塑料网。这些配件都没有经过实验测试，以验证它们是否减少吸烟者接触有害物质或减少他们因烟草引起疾病和死亡的风险。

　　烟斗和烟草的市场营销增强了水烟低有害性的误解。例如，在世界上几个地区销售的一个著名水烟品牌，在其标签上声称"0.5%烟碱和0%焦油"。也有其他品牌声称自己的产品"天然"或"无化学添加"。流行的广告中演示了由椰子或菠萝制成的水烟。一个广告声称，在其产品生产中没有砍掉一棵树。与通常带有强制性健康警示的卷烟包装不同，水烟烟草制品通常销售时没有健康警示。

　　尽管20世纪90年代的中东地区主要是老年男子在抽吸水烟，但是，水烟迅速在年轻人之中流行开来。这一趋势始于中东，并蔓延到许多国家和大洲的大学和中学。在传统水烟使用地区以外的水烟流行度日益增加，反映了国际水烟工业的发展。超过60个国家参与的国际水烟博览会[2]，展现了水烟、水烟烟草和类似产品的最新发展。这些展会的发展反映了人们对水烟产品需求的变化，自2013年设立以来，参观者和参展商不断增加。

2　http://hookahfair.com/index.php/en

5. 水烟流行性增加和发展蔓延的因素

　　一种像抽吸水烟这样的成瘾行为在全球广泛流行，很难确认其所有因素。除非通过有效的政策和法规进行抵制，否则令人上瘾的行为往往会逐渐蔓延。本咨询说明关注了水烟的特点及其在全球迅速蔓延的自身和外部综合因素。这些因素包括：调味烟草的引入，咖啡馆和餐饮文化带来的社会接受度，大众传播和社交媒体的发展，以及针对水烟的政策和法规的匮乏。

5.1　调味烟草（"maassel"）的引入

　　第一次生产出加糖调味烟草（俗称"maassel"）的确切时间无从考证，但早在 20 世纪 90 年代初，它已经在中东地区使用了 [8]。间接证据表明 20 世纪 90 年代初"maassel"的生产与中东地区水烟吸烟者人数的激增之间存在时间上的关联 [8]。"maassel"通常是由烟草混合糖浆、甘油和水果香精发酵，生产出一种湿润、柔软的混合物。在"maassel"之前，大多数水烟吸烟者使用某些形式的自制生烟草（例如，将其碾碎，与水混合，然后挤压成型）。通常这种方法制作的烟产生强烈而刺激的烟气，不像"maassel"的烟气柔和而芳香 [9]。回顾这段历史，"maassel"对于水烟来说，相当于使卷烟得以大规模生产和销售的 Bonsack 机*。"maassel"的工业化和商

---

　　* Bonsack 是最早的卷烟机。——译注

业化及其日益增长的可得性和多样性吸引了年轻人，通过互联网开辟了更广阔的市场，并简化了水烟的生产过程[9]。

来自世界各地的数据显示，对于大多数水烟吸烟者，尤其是年轻人[8-11]，"maassel"是首选的水烟烟草。例如，在2010年美国北卡罗来纳州8所大学3447名学生中进行的调查中，有90%曾经使用水烟的学生使用过"maassel"[11]。许多水烟吸烟者对"maassel"感兴趣是因为它的香味、柔和的烟气及各种各样的口感[12]。

5.2　咖啡馆和餐馆文化带来的社会接受度

抽吸水烟已经在社会层面得到很好的表征[9-14]。许多水烟吸烟者在朋友和家庭聚会中进行这项活动，这成为社会或家庭聚会的核心组成部分[9,10,15,16]。共用同一支水烟也成为公认的、普遍的做法，尤其是在年轻人当中[9,10,17]。人们抽吸水烟会在相对较低的抽吸频率下持续一个小时或更长时间，这有利于发挥其社交功能，特别是在咖啡馆这样的地方。水烟的这些特点恰逢中东地区及至全球年轻人的咖啡馆文化蓬勃繁荣[12]。在这方面的一个里程碑式的事件是20世纪90年代"斋月帐篷盛宴"的出现，这是一种特殊的方式，为斋月期间的穆斯林提供了一个社交场所。特别是年轻人在开戒之后的傍晚聚集在一起，抽吸水烟成了这些聚会中最精华的部分[18]。水烟为吸烟者（斋戒期间禁止吸烟）提供烟碱，成为斋月期间最活跃的社会生活，使吸烟者在严苛的斋戒之后体验长时间的感官放纵。

随着水烟赢得地中海东部地区以外的游客和年轻人的青睐，这个地区的移民将水烟咖啡馆和水烟餐馆开到了世界各地。这些咖啡馆和餐馆有自己的经营方式，此后水烟咖啡馆开始在世界大多数城市的中心城区营业，很大程度上得益于对这种烟草使用的监管体系的薄弱或缺失。例如在美国，水烟咖啡馆在过去十年里数量激增，而且通常开在大学校园旁边[17]。一份对美国 8 所大学 3770 名学生的调查发现，这些学生抽吸水烟与大学校园周围方圆 10 英里（16 km）范围内存在的水烟咖啡馆或餐馆有关[19]。

5.3　大众传播和社交媒体的发展

如果没有全球通信和网络系统，像中东地区抽吸水烟这样的地域趋势，将会保持其地域性，或以较慢速度传播。水烟的迅速传播得益于两项技术的发展。第一项出现在 20 世纪 90 年代，不受管制的、价格低廉、使用广泛的卫星电视覆盖了整个中东地区。结果，卫星电视迅速成为大众娱乐的选择，新的卫星频道不断推出，越来越多的节目间隙时间需要被填满。跟水烟有关的社会活动（如"斋月帐篷盛宴"）很快利用这些间隙时间传遍整个地区[18]。

有可能导致水烟在青少年和受过良好教育人群中越来越受欢迎的第二项技术变革是互联网。在水烟从中东地区传播到对这种烟草使用方式知之甚少甚至一无所知的地区的过程中，互联网功不可没。最近的一项研究比较了 2004~2013 年澳大利亚、加拿大、英国和美国用搜索引擎检索"水烟"和"电子烟"的趋势。研究表明，在这一时期，全部 4 个国家基于互联网的对"水烟"的检索量都稳步上升，在澳大利亚、加拿大和美国，与电子烟相比，对"水烟"的检索更为频繁，检索量的最高值出现在美国（图 2）[20]。

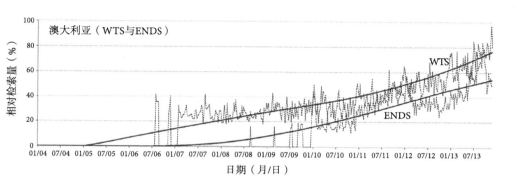

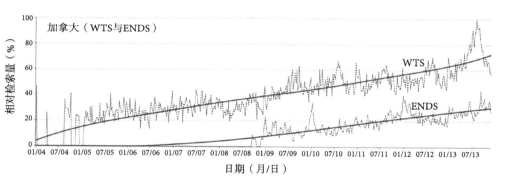

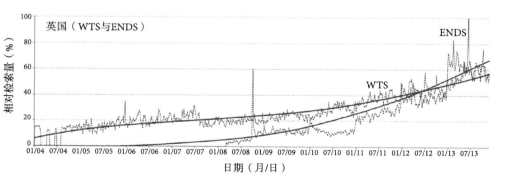

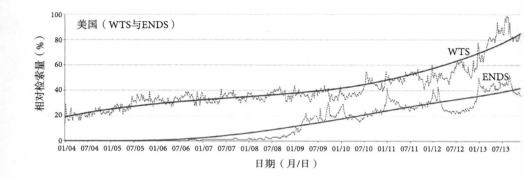

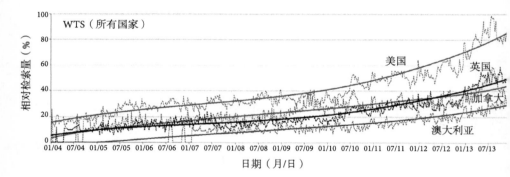

图 2　澳大利亚、加拿大、英国和美国对"水烟"和"电子烟"的互联网检索[20]
WTS：水烟抽吸；ENDS：电子烟碱传输系统（俗称"电子烟"）

　　在线检索最多的是家庭使用的水烟产品，其次是水烟咖啡馆和水烟休息室。基本不受管制的互联网使得水烟推广者绕开了大部分的广告禁令，获得了年轻人及受过良好教育人群这些首选客户资源。在对美国 144 个水烟网站进行分析后发现，只有 4% 的网站张贴了烟草相关的健康警示[21]。一个对卷烟相关和水烟相关 YouTube 视频的相似分析表明，用户上传的水烟相关视频关于吸烟对健康负面影响的认识要比卷烟相关视频少。事实上，92% 的水烟相关视频从正面描述水烟抽吸，而只有 24% 的卷烟相关视频对吸烟持肯定态度[22]。互联网和社交媒体上的大部分宣传都被描绘成相关利益集团的阵线，实际上却是水烟销售者的伪装（例如 www.hookahblogger.tumblr.com/ 和 www.hookah-shisha.com/hookahlove/)[21-23]。

5.4 针对水烟的政策和法规的匮乏

尽管许多国家在降低卷烟抽吸的公众健康政策方面成效显著，但水烟抽吸却因缺乏像卷烟那样严格的烟草控制政策和法规而依然盛行。例如，许多发达国家的水烟场所和水烟产品不受烟草控制政策的制约，而烟草相关控制政策的执行力欠缺是发展中国家的主要问题。这导致了水烟场馆遍布世界各地[14, 24]。

全球的卷烟包装尺寸和包装材料都基本统一，水烟则不同。水烟的形状和尺寸各异，不易携带，由多个部件组成，常常多人共用，并涉及不同的利益相关方。因此，许多政策相关的要素必须专门为水烟定制[25]。例如，一个典型的水烟使用者在公共场所看不到烟草包装及与烟草使用、木炭燃烧或疾病传播有关的健康风险警示[9, 26, 27]。为了解决这个问题，土耳其已经将警示标签扩展到水烟瓶或水烟壶上，要求在水烟瓶两侧的警示应覆盖表面积的 65%[2]。

尽管大多数基于价格的政策有效缩减了卷烟的需求量[28, 29]，但提高 "maassel" 的价格可能不会有同样的效果，特别是在咖啡馆或餐厅，那里的烟草在总利润率中所占比重很小[14]。因为任何人都可以利用相对便宜的原料自制"maassel"[3]，所以相对于卷烟，水烟消费人群对价格不太敏感。此外，调味被认为是吸引年轻人的主要因素，但在烟草中使用香料的禁令还没有适用于水烟产品。

对推动水烟全球传播的因素的概括基于对不同来源的各种证据的收敛性分析。显然这样概括的准确性很有限，但其目的是进一步了解全球水烟迅速传播的动态，从而控制其传播[12]。

3　http://www.thehookahlounge.org/how-to-make-your-own-shisha/（2014 年 7 月 5 日访问）

6. 水烟抽吸的区域模式和全球模式

抽吸水烟传统上与地中海东部地区、东南亚和北非相关[30-32]。然而,水烟的使用正在全球范围增加[1, 31, 33-37],特别是在中学生[31, 38-46]和大学生中间[33, 47, 4]。许多国家并不专门监测水烟;然而,对不同群体和子群体水烟流行性的系统研究显示了惊人的数字,特别是在中东裔的中学生和大学生中[31]。

一些流行性研究表明,在所有 WHO 地区,使用水烟的青少年、成年男性和成年女性都在增加。根据全球 11~15 岁青少年烟草使用情况调查,在 100 个被调查站点中,有 34 个卷烟以外的烟草制品的使用量在增加,这在很大程度上是因为水烟使用量的增加。在报告数据的国家中,水烟流行率为 6%~34%[38]。尽管没有广泛获得国家代表性的成人水烟使用数据,但全球成人烟草使用调查显示,水烟抽吸正在以前不使用这种烟草的国家兴起[34]。本章我们介绍 WHO 六大地区的水烟使用流行情况。

6.1 非 洲 地 区

关于水烟在非洲使用情况的研究有限。在南非的学生中开展了三项实证研究。在第一项研究中,约翰内斯堡一个贫困城市社区有 60% 的高中生曾经使用过水烟,而其中 20% 每天使用[49]。第二项研究发现,在比勒陀利亚的医学生中,19% 的受访者曾经使用过水烟[50]。

在西开普的大学生中进行的第三项研究中，40% 的受访者当前正在使用水烟，其中 70% 每天使用[51]。近一半（48%）的使用者认为抽吸水烟的有害影响被夸大了。青少年将抽吸水烟作为一种社会经验，并认为这种行为和全球化相吻合。

2012 年，在尼日利亚开展的全球成人烟草使用调查中发现[52]，整个 15 岁以上年龄群体中，当前使用非卷烟类烟草制品的比例非常低（总共 0.8%，其中男性 1.6%，女性 0.1%）。尽管缺乏该地区其他国家的相关实验证据 4，但阿尔及利亚、埃塞俄比亚、肯尼亚、尼日利亚、苏丹、乌干达和坦桑尼亚[53] 的坊间证据表明，各大城市中心的时尚水烟酒吧数量激增，其消费人群主要是年轻人和商界人士。

6.2 美 洲 地 区

人们已经对加拿大和美国的水烟抽吸情况进行了一些研究，但对拉丁美洲国家的研究较少。加拿大的一项研究表明，2006~2010 年间，使用水烟的青少年人数增加了 2.6%[54]。随着近些年青少年抽吸卷烟的数量大幅下降，水烟的增长趋势就尤为明显。在美国，有关成年人（年龄在 18 岁以上）的最新数据显示，0.5% 的人每天或每几天抽吸水烟，每天、每几天使用或偶尔抽吸水烟的人总共 3.9%，而每天、每几天或偶尔抽吸水烟的人中，18~24 岁年龄段达 18.2%。

美国的一项全国性研究[56] 获得了 104 434 名大学生使用卷烟、水烟和雪茄的完整资料，其中 8733 人（8.4%）是当前的水烟使用者。

---

4 本咨询说明发布时尚未获取使用喀麦隆、塞内加尔和乌干达关于水烟抽吸的全球成人烟草使用调查结果

在这之中，4492 人（51.4%）没有使用卷烟，3609 人（41.3%）没有使用其他形式的烟草。在全部 104 434 名调查对象中，31 749 人（30.4%）曾经使用水烟，其中 9423 人（29.7%）从未使用过卷烟，6198 人（19.5%）从未使用过任何其他烟草。因此，继卷烟之后，水烟成了最常见的烟草消费方式。未成年人过去一个月抽吸水烟的比例为 2.6%，以任何方式使用烟草的比例为 7.3%。研究者得出结论："几乎每 5 名未成年人中就有 1 名在高中毕业之前尝试水烟。"一项针对高中生的国家代表性研究表明，过去一年，这些高中生中有 18% 使用水烟；那些具有较高社会经济地位的人群正处在水烟抽吸的风险之中[57]。

虽然已发表的文献有限，但拉丁美洲地区并没有呈现同样严重的水烟抽吸情况。全球成人烟草调查表明，巴西（2008 年）、墨西哥（2009 年）、巴拉圭（2010 年）及阿根廷（2012 年）抽吸水烟的比例都很低，这四个国家总共才不到 0.2%[34, 58]。青少年的比例同样不高。

6.3 地中海东部地区

地中海东部地区（包括中东地区和北非地区的国家）的水烟使用者比例全世界最高[59]，尤其是青少年[30-32, 60]。2008~2010 年对该地区青少年吸烟情况的纵向研究发现，在随访的 2 年内，抽吸水烟的人数增加了 40%（从 13.3% 增加到 18.9%，$p<0.01$）[61]。在该地区不同国家对 13~15 岁年龄段在校学生的代表性研究中，抽吸水烟者的比例在 9%~15%[62]。在这些研究中，水烟抽吸者的比例实际上高于卷烟抽吸者。全球青少年烟草使用调查显示，在该地区所有 17 个国家[38]

的 13~15 岁年龄段的青少年中，使用其他形式烟草制品（主要是水烟）的人数要高于使用卷烟的人数。

全球成人烟草使用调查获得了埃及（2009 年）[63] 和卡塔尔（2013 年）[64] 的成年人数据。在 15 岁以上年龄段，埃及有 6.2% 的男性和 0.3% 的女性使用水烟，卡塔尔有 4.9% 的男性和 1.6% 的女生使用水烟。在埃及，抽吸水烟的男性往往年龄较大（40~54 岁），生活在偏远地区，且受教育程度较低，这与以往的研究结果一致，反映了埃及抽吸水烟的传统 [34]。

6.4 欧洲地区

根据全球成人烟草使用调查，15 岁以上人群当前和日常抽吸水烟者少于抽吸卷烟者。抽吸水烟人数比例最高的是俄罗斯（2009 年，4.4%），其次是土耳其（2008 年，4.0%）、乌克兰（2010 年，3.2%）和罗马尼亚（2011 年，0.3% ）[34, 65]。在这些国家，水烟使用者年轻（18~24 岁），居住在城市地区，受过良好教育，且往往是偶尔而不是每天都抽吸水烟 [34]。

根据 2012 年欧洲联盟 28 个成员国 15 岁以上人群吸烟情况及对烟草态度的民意调查报告（Eurobarometer report）[35]，16% 的受访者称，他们至少尝试过一次水烟，这比 2009 年的调查结果要高。水烟最普及的国家是拉脱维亚（42%）、爱沙尼亚（37%）和立陶宛（36%），水烟使用最少的国家是爱尔兰（5%）、葡萄牙（5%）、马耳他（8%）和西班牙（8%）。奥地利、捷克和卢森堡的水烟用量增长幅度最大，而瑞典的跌幅最大。一般来说，年轻的男性受访者和学生的水烟使用量最大。

较小规模的研究也显示，欧洲越来越多的人使用水烟。在英国，大学生使用水烟的比例为 8%~11%，而中学生为 8%[47, 66, 67]。在法国，对 920 名高中学生（平均年龄 18 岁）的研究发现，有 40% 的受访者表示尝试过除卷烟以外的其他烟草制品，包括水烟[68]。在对爱沙尼亚的 13 826 名学生（11~15 岁）的全国性研究中，25% 的男孩和 16% 的女孩使用过水烟[69]。在以色列的一项对中学生的研究中，22% 每周都使用水烟[70]。以色列的其他研究也显示，中学生（<18 岁）的水烟使用率很高[71, 72]，达到 40%[73]。

6.5　东南亚地区

全球成人烟草使用调查收集了 2008~2011 年孟加拉国和泰国（2009 年）、印度（2010 年）以及印度尼西亚（2011 年）的水烟使用数据[34, 74]。男性使用水烟比例最高的是孟加拉国（1.3%），其次是印度（1.1%），印度尼西亚（0.3%）和泰国（0.03%）；女性使用水烟比例最高的是印度（0.6%），其次是孟加拉国（0.2%），泰国（0.01%）和印度尼西亚（0.0%）。印度的水烟抽吸者中，50 岁以上年龄段的人数明显高于 30 岁以下年龄段（分别为 2.0% 和 0.3%），生活在偏远地区的多于生活在城市地区的（分别为 1.1% 和 0.0%），受教育程度低的多于受教育程度高的（分别为 1.4% 和 0.0%），同时抽吸卷烟的多于不抽吸卷烟的（分别为 5.6% 和 0.6%）[75]。

没有获得该地区其他国家的水烟抽吸流行性实验数据；然而，来自报纸和互联网的坊间证据显示，水烟酒吧和水烟餐馆越来越普遍，且经常光顾的大多是年轻人。

6.6　西太平洋地区

在亚洲，吸食烟草从"bong"水烟[5]（图3）开始，经历了漫长的历史过程。"bong"水烟与传统的阿拉伯水烟[34]不同，通常不包括在水烟抽吸研究中。"bong"水烟可由竹子、金属或玻璃制成，在中国、老挝、缅甸和越南等国家使用。常有一种误解认为"bong"水烟的危害性低于地中海东部地区的水烟[76]。

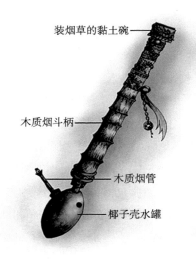

装烟草的黏土碗

木质烟斗柄

木质烟管

椰子壳水罐

图3　中国"bong"水烟

_____

5　"bong"与中东地区使用的水烟略微不同：它不需要使用木炭，可能降低了一氧化碳暴露

对比了全球 13 个国家，15 岁以上年龄段男性使用水烟的比例最高的是越南（2010 年，13.0%），高于埃及（2009 年，6.2%）和土耳其（2008 年，4.0%）[34]。在越南，抽吸水烟比例最高的是年龄较大（40~54岁）、生活在偏远地区以及受教育程度较低的人群。越南女性使用水烟的比例非常低（0.2%）。

全球成人烟草使用调查显示，在 15 岁以上年龄段，中国（2010年）只有 0.65% 的男性和 0.08% 的女性使用水烟，马来西亚（2011 年）有 1.0% 的男生和 0.1% 的女性使用水烟[77]。

传统的"bong"水烟倾向于在年长、偏远地区及受教育程度较低的男性使用。然而，有一些坊间证据表明，许多传统的中东水烟咖啡馆正在该地区的城市开放，并且越来越普遍，水烟抽吸情况应当受到监控。上述没有对传统的地中海东部地区水烟和"bong"水烟进行调查。

7. 水烟烟气有害成分的健康影响

由于燃烧的木炭通常用作水烟的热源，所以烟气中含有从炭和烟草制品（包括调味剂）排出的有害物质。因此，木炭和烟草的组成都会影响烟气的有害成分。

过去十年里，实验室研究使用现代分析方法和可靠的机械化烟气产生与采样方案，已经开始阐明水烟的有害成分。已鉴定出许多致癌物和有害物质，如烟草特有亚硝胺、多环芳烃（PAH，如苯并[a]芘、蒽）、挥发性醛（如甲醛、乙醛、丙烯醛）、苯、一氧化氮和重金属（砷、铬、铅）。木炭会产生高浓度的一氧化碳（CO）和致癌物 PAH[2]。其中一些化学物质被国际癌症研究机构（IARC）列为人体致癌物 [78]。据 2014 年的报道，暴露于水烟烟气的人会由于吸入苯而有罹患白血病的风险 [79]。

影响水烟烟气气溶胶有害性的其他因素还包括抽吸模式（即抽吸口数，每口的抽吸量、持续时间，以及两口抽吸之间的时间间隔）和水烟的设计与制造。尽管已经在水烟标准化方面做过一些尝试，但水烟仍未标准化，其形式多种多样，包括水碗之上水烟头的空间容量以及供使用者吸入烟气的软管的孔隙率各不相同。通过改变稀释效果和燃烧条件，不同的软管孔隙度可以极大地影响有害物质含量 [80]。

因此，已发表的关于水烟烟气有害成分的研究报告针对木炭和烟草的具体组合以及特定的水烟特征和抽吸参数。与卷烟烟气一样，水烟烟气的有害物质含量差别很大。然而，迄今为止的所有研究表明，在一段典型的水烟使用周期内，使用者会吸入大剂量的有害物质（相当于从低于一支卷烟到数十支卷烟）（图 4）。对卷烟使用者来说，这些有害物质与成瘾、心肺疾病及癌症有关；对水烟使用者来说，如果这些有害物质的吸收量达到一定程度，也会导致相同的结果。

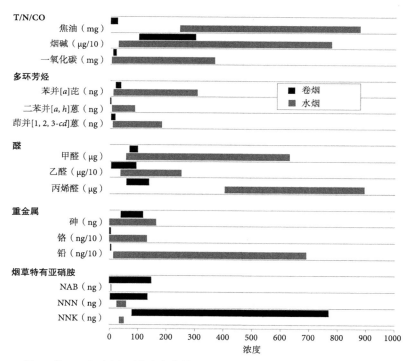

图 4　使用 1 小时水烟（灰色）和抽吸 1 支卷烟（黑色）产生的有害物质浓度

NAB：N- 亚硝基假木贼碱；NNN：N- 亚硝基降烟碱；NNK：4-(N- 甲基亚硝胺基)-1-(3- 吡啶基)-1- 丁酮

卷烟数据来自 Apsley 等 [81] 和 Jenkins 等 [82]；水烟数据来自 Monzer 等 [83]，Schubert 等 [84] 和 Shihadeh[85]

水烟产品中的烟碱是水烟潜在依赖性（致瘾性）的原因。配备 1.5 倍点燃木炭盘的水烟头，在一个 10 g "maassel" 烟草的抽吸过程中，主流烟气中烟碱释放量为 2.94 mg，焦油释放量为 802 mg，CO 释放量为 145 mg[2]。

7.1　水烟使用者的有害成分摄入

水烟烟气分析清楚地表明其含有大量的有害成分，但是并未反映使用者是否显著吸收了这些有害成分。因此，评估水烟使用潜在危害的另一个调查方向是研究使用者血液和尿液中有害成分暴露的生物标志物。这类研究已经调研了 CO、烟碱、PAH 或烟草特有亚硝胺的急性暴露、多日暴露以及长期暴露[86-91]。抽吸水烟会导致所有这些化合物的显著暴露，与卷烟抽吸者相比，水烟使用者的 CO 暴露量极显著升高，PAH 暴露量显著升高，烟碱暴露量类似，烟草特有亚硝胺暴露量显著较低[87,91]。不同研究的结果是一致的，反映了水烟和卷烟的烟气有害成分含量分析发现的模式差异。尽管水烟烟气与卷烟烟气中烟碱含量差不多，但与卷烟烟气相比，水烟烟气中含有更多的 CO，更多的 PAH 和较少的烟草特有亚硝胺。对水烟使用者和卷烟使用者血液和尿液中暴露生物标志物的比较也反映了这个结果。

7.2　使用水烟的急性生理和健康影响

水烟对呼吸系统、心血管系统、口腔和牙齿具有不良影响，且长期使用水烟者慢性阻塞性肺疾病和牙周病的患病率较高[2, 92]。

由于 CO 中毒继发形成碳氧血红蛋白，阻碍血液向身体各器官（包括大脑）传输足够的氧气，因此释放高浓度的 CO 会导致某些吸烟者昏厥 [2]。水烟使用者急性 CO 中毒事件已被报道过 [93, 94]，几项临床对照研究也报道了急性反应。其中一些急性反应，如心率加快，血压升高，与已知的烟碱反应一致 [95-97]。另外一些急性心血管的不良反应，如压力反射控制受损 [98] 和心脏自主神经功能障碍 [87, 88] 也得以发现，并且发现与烟碱含量无关。抽吸水烟似乎还会损害肺功能和运动机能 [99]，并引起炎症生物标志物的变化 [96]。这些反应与水烟烟气不仅传输生理活性剂量的烟碱而且还有其他有害成分的观点一致，表明长期使用水烟从长远来看可能会引发疾病。

7.3 二手水烟烟气

对照实验室试验箱 [100,101] 和水烟使用环境中大气颗粒物测试结果 [102-104] 显示，直接从水烟释放到周围环境中的二手烟气也含有有害成分。总体而言，这些研究表明抽吸水烟导致 CO、醛、PAH、超细颗粒物和可吸入颗粒物的大量释放。在建筑物内如果只使用水烟，其可吸入颗粒物浓度往往要比只抽吸卷烟高 [102, 103]。同样抽吸 1 小时，水烟释放的 CO、PAH 和挥发性醛的浓度要高于卷烟 [105]。此外，无烟草配方制备的水烟直接释放的有害成分等于或高于用烟草制备的水烟。因此，除了烟碱，无烟草水烟制品的烟气具有与含烟草水烟制品相同的有害成分释放量和生物活性 [103]。这些研究表明，水烟抽吸应当被纳入旨在减少二手烟暴露的所有规定。

7.4　长期健康影响

一份对抽吸水烟的健康影响的系统综述表明，抽吸水烟与肺癌、牙周病和低出生体重显著相关[106]。当时（2010 年）的证据不足以排除或证实抽吸水烟与其他疾病（包括其他类型的癌症）有关。那份综述之后，又发表了 20 多项新的相关研究，这些研究构成了证据基础，有助于更好地了解抽吸水烟对健康的影响，以下进行详述。

截至 2014 年 6 月的现有证据表明，抽吸水烟可能与以下类型的癌症有关：口腔癌，比值比*为 4，基于在印度和也门开展的两项横向研究[107, 108]；食道癌，比值比为 2.65，基于在伊朗和克什米尔地区开展的三项病例 - 对照研究[109-111]；以及肺癌，比值比为 2.12，基于在中国[6]、印度和突尼斯开展的六项研究[112-117]。

在伊朗开展的一项病例 - 对照研究和一项前瞻性队列研究表明，抽吸水烟还可能与胃癌有关[118, 119]；在埃及开展的两项病例 - 对照研究表明抽吸水烟与膀胱癌有关[120, 121]。在过去 5 年间，获得了抽吸水烟与呼吸道疾病（主要是慢性支气管炎）有关的重要证据。对来自中东地区和北非地区的五项研究的数据进行的荟萃分析显示，合并的比值比约为 2[122-126]。此外，抽吸卷烟和抽吸水烟对慢性阻塞性肺病具有协同效应[127]。一项关于中国抽吸水烟的研究显示，水烟抽吸

---

　　*　在病例 - 对照研究中，比值比（odds ratio，OR）指病例组暴露人数与非暴露人数的比值除以对照组暴露人数与非暴露人数的比值，是分析疾病与暴露因素关联程度的指标。——译注

　　6　中国水烟和图 1 所示的水烟有所不同。见图 3

者和暴露于二手水烟烟气的妇女罹患慢性阻塞性肺病的风险显著增加（比值比 >10）[76]。重要的是，这种疾病通常与肺癌相关[128]。

在心血管疾病方面，一项覆盖黎巴嫩 4 家医院 1210 名患者的研究中，校正了人口统计学因素以及冠心病的个体特征和风险（抽吸卷烟、饮酒、缺乏体育锻炼、糖尿病、高血压、高血脂和冠心病家族史）之后得出，抽吸水烟 40 年以上者血管严重阻塞的发病率（70%）比非吸烟者高 3 倍（比值比 2.95；95% 置信区间，1.04~8.33）[129]。另一项在孟加拉国进行的大型前瞻性研究表明，抽吸水烟导致缺血性心脏病和中风引起的死亡率增加 20%[130]。伊朗的一项横向研究关于抽吸水烟和心脏病之间的关联没有给出确凿的证据，但显示了剂量 - 效应关系（即高暴露带来高风险），使得这种关联更具可能性[131]。一些研究已经讨论了替代结果，诸如心血管造影结果的严重程度，其结果与上述研究结果一致[129, 132]。

在埃及进行的三项横向研究没有表明水烟使用与丙型肝炎病毒感染有关[133-135]。虽然有病例报告水烟抽吸与结核病有关[27, 136, 137]，但目前还没有说明这种关联的正式研究报告发表。

有两项研究评估了水烟烟草抽吸与生活质量之间的关系。一项在黎巴嫩开展的全国横向研究中没有发现水烟抽吸与 "呼吸生活质量" 7[138] 相关的确凿证据，而在伊朗的一项类似研究发现，水烟抽吸者的健康相关生活质量较差[139]。

抽吸水烟还会造成许多其他后果。在黎巴嫩进行的两次回顾性队列研究和在伊朗进行的一项病例 - 对照研究发现抽吸水烟与低出

7　呼吸生活质量的显著预测因子，按重要性递减的顺序如下：抽吸卷烟的累积数量，较大的年龄，家庭中至少有一个吸烟者，受教育程度低，女性，家庭使用燃油取暖，水烟烟气的累积剂量，家庭使用暖风取暖，同事中至少有一个吸烟者

生体重之间存在关联，比值比约为 2[140-142]。埃及的一项队列研究和沙特阿拉伯的四项横向研究均显示水烟抽吸与牙周病之间存在统计学显著关联[143-147]。

此外还有一些关于水烟使用和其他健康影响之间关联的单独报告。黎巴嫩的一项横向研究发现抽吸水烟与常年性鼻炎之间存在联系[148]；埃及的一项研究表明水烟抽吸与男性不育有关[49]；伊朗的一项大型横向研究表明水烟抽吸与胃食管反流病有关联[149]；一项美国大学生的全国调查发现，抽吸水烟和心理健康情况较差之间存在中度的显著关联[150]。

7.5　水烟致瘾性

抽吸水烟的一个主要特点是其独特的使用方式[7]。特别是在年轻人中，抽吸水烟经常在朋友聚会或家族聚会中被作为集体的消遣。一个水烟抽吸周期平均 1 小时，它有限的可获得性或者说流动性使得间歇性使用成为其主要模式[7]。此外，还存在水具有过滤效果的常见误解。这些特征表明为什么许多水烟抽吸者声称它不像卷烟那样使人上瘾[151]。目前尚不知晓抽吸水烟是否与使用同等水平的卷烟一样令人上瘾，但是有证据表明，抽吸水烟成瘾的证据正在逐渐累加并越来越明显。

1997 年，Macaron 及其同事通过检测尿液中的可替宁，首次揭示了水烟抽吸者的烟碱暴露情况[152]；此后的重复实验获得了同样的结果。例如，在叙利亚烟草研究中心近期的一项实验室研究中，已经禁烟 24 小时的水烟抽吸者在临床实验室抽吸水烟 1 个周期，抽取他们的静脉血液用于随后的烟碱分析。抽吸水烟导致血浆烟碱水平升高约 5 倍（从抽吸前的 3.07 ng/mL ± 3.05 ng/mL 到抽吸后的 15.7 ng/mL ± 8.7 ng/mL；$p<0.001$）[153]。在另一项研究中，将水烟使用者和卷烟使用者的烟碱暴露在双因素交叉设计下进行了比较（即如果第一个周期抽吸水烟，则第二个周期抽吸卷烟，反之亦然）。虽然血浆烟碱水平峰值在两种条件下没有差异，但是暴露动力学和烟碱的累积剂量是不同的，与卷烟抽吸者相比，水烟抽吸者上升缓慢，持续时间较长，累积暴露量较大（图 5）[154]。

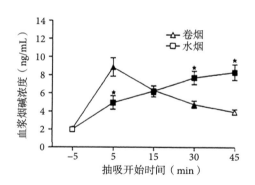

图 5 31 名水烟抽吸者（三角形）和卷烟抽吸者（正方形）在一个实验室周期中血浆烟碱浓度均值（± 平均标准误差）

对水烟和卷烟均未限制时间，水烟可抽吸 45 min，卷烟抽吸约 5 min。实心符号表示与基线（时间为 0）存在显著差异，星号（*）表示两因素之间存在显著差异（$p<0.001$）

除了烟碱介导成瘾的神经药理学方面，行为学研究也表明水烟抽吸者的依赖性，例如失败的戒烟尝试，对水烟着迷的自我感觉，随着时间的推移使用升级，为确保获取而调整行为，以及戒除不成功并继续使用[33]。例如，叙利亚阿勒颇的一项 268 名水烟使用者的随机抽样中，28% 的人想戒除，59% 的人在过去一年里有过失败的戒烟尝试。对戒烟能力的信念与感知到的依赖性存在负相关关系 [155]。这一经验已在标准化的实验室环境中得到证实，水烟抽吸者禁烟 24 小时后被带到叙利亚烟草研究中心的临床实验室随意抽吸水烟，在抽吸前后对他们的主观戒断和主观渴求进行测量。结果表明，抽烟的冲动、焦躁、渴求及其他戒断症状在抽吸前很强烈，但抽吸后显著减轻，而感觉晕眩或头晕等烟碱的直接反应则呈现相反的趋势 [156]。

与水烟使用者的面谈揭示了更多这种抽吸形式成瘾性的信息。例如，一项定性研究给出了来自水烟抽吸者的几段有趣的话："我年轻的时候就开始吸烟（水烟）了，我知道它的副作用，也知道它对我的肺做了什么。我上个楼梯都会喘。但我无法（戒掉它），因为我对它上瘾了，我不介意不再抽它，但我不能。""我喜欢掌控一切，但是 narghile（水烟）完全控制着我。这让我很烦。我的快乐就与 narghile 有关。它是享受美好时光不可或缺的……""我通常每天抽吸一次，但有时抽得更多。因为即使我已经吸过了，看到或闻到 narghile 仍会让我觉得我需要再次抽烟，我确实经常抽烟。"[157]这些说法符合抽吸水烟的烟草和烟碱依赖性与抽吸卷烟一致的观点。

虽然许多关于水烟依赖的指标在抽吸卷烟中也存在，但有充分的理由让我们相信，水烟的独特特征会影响使用者烟草依赖的发展和表现。水烟共享的社会层面和有限的可获得性特点通常未被纳入烟草依赖的传统模型 [7]。此外，因为水烟通常可被重复使用，所以相对于买一包卷烟来说，寻找一副水烟的行为甚至可以说是一件"里程碑"式的大事。然而，目前对水烟依赖性的研究还依靠来自卷烟相关文献的模型和方法，这可能导致对抽吸水烟潜在致瘾性的不充分甚至错误的判断。例如，在醒来的最初 30 分钟内渴求吸烟，这是预测卷烟吸烟者烟草依赖性的有力证据，最近的一篇文献基于缺乏这一证据而对抽吸水烟的成瘾性进行了质疑 [158]。鉴于抽吸水烟的已知模式，即在轻松氛围和社会环境中进行较长的抽吸过程，这种质疑毫无道理。大约十年前，水烟专家就对使用卷烟专用的量表或条目(例如在醒来的最初30分钟内吸烟)来评估水烟依赖性提出了警告，因为已知的水烟使用模式与卷烟不同 [159]。

抽吸水烟的潜在致瘾性证据促使人们努力开发其烟草依赖的特定测量方法。其中一项开拓的方法是黎巴嫩水烟依赖量表 [160]。这个量表并不是基于水烟抽吸者的数据，而是源于烟碱依赖的 Fager-ström 量表和《精神疾病诊断与统计手册》(第 4 次修订版)，已经在若干研究中用以测量水烟使用者的依赖性 [161-163]。即便有了说明，水烟抽吸者的烟草依赖因为其独有的特点，那些来自卷烟相关文献的模型或仪器仍不被认可。某些特点可能影响了水烟抽吸者成瘾发展的所有阶段。因此，虽然水烟的特异性气味和声音可能会吸引新的使用者并加强既定吸烟者的使用，但是确保获取的行为适应可能意味着更进一步的依赖。每日抽吸者认为自己已经水烟成瘾，会进行更彻底的行为适应，以确保水烟的可获得性，如购置自己的水烟，选择有水烟的咖啡馆 [37]。

已有一些研究阐述了水烟特异性特征在吸引新的抽吸者及强化使用中的作用 [162]。例如，最近在黎巴嫩进行的一项定性研究支持了水烟的气味、声音和口感等特征吸引年轻人这个观点 [18]。具体来说，水烟烟草 "maassel" 的口感和气味被一些人列为尝试水烟并最终成瘾的主要原因："我父母过去常常坐下来抽吸水烟……那时，我被它好闻的气味吸引了。"甚至在公共场所，水烟的气味也能成为一些人开始抽吸的动因："当你到达一家咖啡馆，从外面闻到水烟的味道，你会说就是它了，你想抽烟。"此外，对地中海东部地区和其他地方的水烟抽吸者的态度和行为的研究，重复验证了水烟体验过程中诸如芳香气味、柔和的口感和冒泡的声音这些特点的影响 [10, 12, 33, 152, 162, 164]。水烟使用的这些独特特征及其相关联的对使用者的诱导，要求基于对水烟抽吸者成瘾的发展和特性以及影响因素的研究证据来制定预防和戒断水烟的全新方法。

7.6　水烟作为抽吸卷烟的桥梁

　　抽吸水烟扩散的另一个令人担忧的方面是它可能阻碍成人吸烟者的戒烟尝试，并且会作为青少年转而抽吸卷烟的途径。一些证据支持了这种可能性。首先，地中海东部地区的戒烟研究表明，一些戒掉卷烟的人转而使用水烟，或许是为了满足他们的渴求并避免戒断反应 [165]。一项临床实验室研究进一步调查了在卷烟戒烟者用水烟替代卷烟的潜在可能，在该项研究中，水烟和卷烟双重使用者在禁烟12小时后，在48小时内参与了两个随机顺序的抽吸过程（水烟或卷烟）。对于这两种烟草使用方法，戒断反应和渴求在过程开始时（吸烟前）都较高，并且在抽吸过程中显著并同等地降低（图6）[166]。

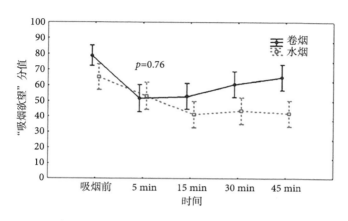

图 6　被禁烟的卷烟和水烟双重使用者"吸烟冲动"项目的平均分值
比较了 5 min 时的重复模型方差分析，$p = 0.8$

　　成人吸烟者的定性研究扩展了这一观察结果，表明卷烟戒断者使用水烟有助于缓解戒断症状，但会增加戒烟失败的可能性。例如，在一项成人水烟和卷烟使用者的定性研究中，一名吸烟者说："我已戒烟（卷烟）6 个多月了。然后，我被邀请抽吸 narghile（水烟）。第二口之后，我要了一支卷烟，我又开始抽吸卷烟了。"[157]

　　虽然这些研究结果表明了水烟替代卷烟以及作为卷烟抽吸的桥梁的可能性，但是关于抽吸水烟导致抽吸卷烟的这种"入门"假设仍在研究中。通常来说，水烟由于其尺寸和耗时的准备过程，相比于卷烟更难被吸烟者获得。这些特征对需要频繁抽吸的成瘾行为来说是一个限制，这就使得从水烟开始烟草使用的年轻人可能转向更容易获得的卷烟，从而更快地缓解他们的烟草依赖[33]。换句话说，可能是依赖性和可获得性之间的平衡决定了水烟使用者可能开始抽吸卷烟。一项以不使用水烟或卷烟的青少年（年龄 13 岁以上）为基准，与鉴于卷烟抽吸未来风险而从不吸烟的人作比较的纵向研究检验了这个假设。水烟抽吸者 12 个月内开始抽吸卷烟的风险是从不吸烟的人的两倍，并且此风险取决于剂量（图 7）[167]。

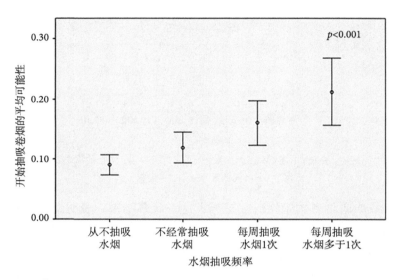

图 7　约旦伊尔比德 2008~2011 年 1454 名未成年人 12 个月内开始卷烟抽吸的平均
预估可能性与上一年水烟抽吸频率之间的关联

这些结果有力支持了抽吸水烟作为卷烟抽吸桥梁的可能性，并支持了更频繁（依赖性更强）的吸烟者更可能转向卷烟的合理性[168]。

综上所述，为了有效地应对水烟依赖性，需要水烟专有模型和检测方法，来获取水烟使用者抽吸史上各方面体验的完整数据。环境因素（例如政策、家庭、文化）和卷烟抽吸在水烟使用传播中所起的作用也需要更清晰的认识。这些认知能够指导水烟特有的预防和干预策略，从而遏制其全球蔓延。

8. 研究需求

　　水烟在全球范围的广泛使用，以及使用者确实 [86, 90] 或可能 [169] 暴露的多种有害成分，为研究与这种烟草使用方式有关的健康风险及预防和治疗方法提供了充足的理由。目前一些研究领域已取得了显著进展，本咨询说明显示，我们在以下方面均有所进展：了解水烟烟草的国家和全球趋势，评价有害成分释放量的方法，吸烟者对有害成分的暴露和吸收，个人抽吸模式，释放量、暴露量和吸收量之间的关系，以及水烟烟气的药理学和毒理学效应。在过去十年里，水烟使用相关研究已经急剧增加，尤其是在德国、约旦、黎巴嫩、英国和美国，但还是需要更多的研究 [170, 171]。然而因为个别研究团体倾向于相对孤立地工作，导致了研究进展缓慢。

　　进行更多水烟烟草方方面面研究 [164, 172] 的反复呼吁已经得到了全球的积极响应，但还有更多工作需要做。需要协调行动来解决下面列出的关键研究需求：

- 所有区域和文化背景下抽吸水烟的类型和模式 [1]；
- 水烟装置和抽吸条件决定烟气的化学和物理性质的程度 [1]；
- 与水烟相关的急性健康影响及患病风险的流行病学研究，包括致癌性、非烟草相关传染病的传播 [1]、呼吸道癌症以及心血管和其他烟草相关疾病的传播，特别是了解使用模式（例如，频率、放置在水烟头和 / 或烟草碗中的成分或原料、群体或个体抽吸过程以及是否共用吸嘴）对疾病风险的影响，还应考虑特殊群体，例如孕妇和育龄妇女；

- 标准化的暴露生物标志物的开发及其效应，例如 DNA 加合物，用以获得水烟烟气对细胞和试验动物的生物效应的补充证据，从而确定水烟烟气是否诱导炎症和氧化应激反应；
- 文化和社会对开始和维持抽吸的影响[1]；
- 抽吸水烟与其他形式烟草的关系，包括替代及抽吸多种产品[1]，以及抽吸水烟作为开始转而使用其他形式烟草的可能性；
- 抽吸水烟与使用包括大麻在内的其他药物之间的关系[1]；
- 与文化相关的预防和戒烟策略的制定[1]；
- 对水烟有效的烟碱和烟草依赖评价方法的制定，同时考虑文化和语言的差异；
- 调味烟草、水烟咖啡馆和其他营销工具、经济因素以及水烟特异性烟草管控措施缺失等对水烟烟草抽吸的全球蔓延的影响程度；
- 非吸烟者的水烟烟草烟气暴露反应，包括健康影响和烟草抽吸的"再归一化"；
- 临床和公共卫生干预对预防和停止抽吸水烟的影响的实验研究；
- 不含烟草或含低浓度烟碱烟草的水烟是否导致依赖；
- 水烟烟草抽吸的表观遗传效应，例如在人呼吸道上皮细胞中；
- 调味剂在促进开始使用，双重使用及继续使用其他类型烟草制品等方面所起的作用及其长期影响；
- 对 WHO 烟草实验室网络（TobLabNet）[8]，根据世界卫生

---

8   http://www.who.int/tobacco/industry/product_regulation/toblabnet/en/

组织《烟草控制框架公约》缔约方大会第六次会议（WHO FCTC COP6）要求 [176]，在 2 年内评估测量卷烟烟气成分及释放物中烟碱 [173]、烟草特有亚硝胺 [174] 和苯并 [a] 芘 [175] 的标准操作规程是否适用于或经调整后适用于水烟烟气 [176]。

9. 科学依据和结论

　　虽然关于抽吸水烟烟草的健康影响的证据基础仍然很少，但现有证据仍然足以证明应采取强有力的控制措施来限制水烟抽吸的传播。如上所述，迄今为止的每一项研究都发现，水烟烟气含有大量的已知在卷烟抽吸者中引发疾病（包括癌症）的有害成分，并且至少其中一些有害成分可被水烟使用者吸入，并因此存在于他们呼出的气体以及血液和尿液中[177]。水烟烟气对细胞和试验动物生物效应的研究提供了补充证据，表明其诱导炎症和氧化应激反应[178]，并为水烟规律性使用者的血管疾病和慢性阻塞性肺疾病的发展提供了可能的机制。这些流行病学研究的结果与毒理学研究的结果一致。逐渐累积的证据表明，抽吸水烟烟草很可能与口腔癌、食道癌和肺癌有关，并可能与胃癌和膀胱癌有关。还有证据表明其与呼吸系统疾病、心血管疾病、牙周病、低出生体重、常年性鼻炎、男性不育、胃食管反流病和精神健康障碍有关[91]。水烟抽吸与肺结核的关联仍存在不确定性。

　　总之，从分子研究到人群研究的所有证据都支持抽吸水烟与抽吸卷烟同样引发疾病（包括成瘾）的结论。虽然相比卷烟烟气，对水烟烟气成分及其生物活性和健康影响的研究较少，但同一科学方法及不同科学方法之间证据的一致性有力说明这一基本结论不会随着更多证据的出现而改变。随着全世界范围水烟使用的增长，必须采取坚决行动，保护公众健康。

10. 政策

  2014 年 10 月 13~18 日在俄罗斯莫斯科举行的世界卫生组织《烟草控制框架公约》（WHO FCTC）第六次缔约方大会上，WHO 受邀根据 WHO FCTC 编写一份关于控制水烟烟草制品使用的策略选择和最优方法的报告，该报告于 2016 年 11 月在第七次缔约方大会上提交[179]。为此，TobReg 提出以下政策建议。

WHO FCTC 条款	专门针对水烟的政策建议
第 5 条	**一般义务。** 即使在具有完善的烟草控制规划的国家，水烟烟草抽吸也可能被忽视或豁免，这是由于在一些国家水烟是新兴的，而在另一些国家有长期的传统存在。关于烟草的立法和条例应当针对所有烟草，而不仅仅局限于卷烟，并应确保在具有较高流行性或流行性越来越高的国家的立法中纳入关于水烟的规定[9]。
第 5.3 条	**商业利益回避。** 近期举办了推广水烟烟草制品及配件的国际展销会[1]。应该对直接或通过第三方拥护或反对法律法规的水烟烟草及其配件公司提出透明度要求。无论烟草公司在水烟制品的生产、分销和零售中发挥什么作用，只要它继续从烟草及其产品中牟取利益或代表其利益，该企业、其同盟和外围组织永远不能被认为是合法的公共卫生合作伙伴或利益相关者。
第 6 条	**降低烟草需求的价格和税收措施。** 由于税收措施已在降低烟草消费方面显示出作用，特别是对年轻人来说，缔约方应针对水烟烟草和水烟产品实施税收和价格措施。
第 8 条	**预防烟草烟暴露。** 因为所有二手烟草烟气都有可能导致死亡、残疾和疾病，所以水烟应与卷烟一样被纳入室内空气清洁政策中。水烟咖啡馆或水烟休息室不应免于室内空气清洁法案。
第 9 条和第 10 条	**烟草制品成分及释放物的管制和披露。** 应实施相关政策以确保水烟烟草纳入需要测试管制烟草成分及释放物的立法中，并进行报告。

---

9 水烟头中含有或不含烟草的水烟

咨询说明：
水烟抽吸——健康影响、研究需求和监管措施

第 11 条 a	**健康声明。**水烟烟草包装和所有水烟部件及配件不得造成对烟草的任何误解，也不得对其使用本身的危害性给出错误的看法。
b	**健康警示。**水烟烟草、产品包装和水烟本身应按照 WHO FCTC 第 11 条要求标有健康警示。
第 12 条	**教育、公众意识和培训。**鉴于抽吸水烟烟草的健康危害的错误信息盛行，缔约方应在更广泛的烟草教育和公众意识方案中纳入专门针对水烟的教育和培训。
第 13 条	**广告、促销和赞助。**依据 WHO FCTC 第 13 条，应全面禁止水烟的广告、促销和赞助。不能进行全面禁止的缔约方应极力限制此类广告、促销和赞助。
第 14 条	**减少烟草需求的措施——关于烟草依赖和戒烟。**根据 WHO FCTC 第 14 条和实施指南中所列措施，缔约方应将抽吸水烟纳入戒烟和治疗烟草依赖的方案中。
第 15 条	**烟草制品的非法贸易。**禁止烟草非法贸易的立法和措施应遵循 WHO FCTC 第 15 条规定的指导方针，并应确保水烟烟草和卷烟以及所有其他形式的烟草一样被包括其中。
第 16 条	**禁止向（或通过）未成年人销售。**根据 WHO FCTC 第 16 条，禁止向未成年人销售所有烟草制品，包括水烟烟草。水烟会所也不例外。
附加条款	**产品设计和信息。**水烟和水烟制品应当受以下条款管制： • 减少有害成分及释放物； • 确保使用的烟碱达到药理学品质； • 降低烟碱急性毒性； • 减少来自木炭加热的 CO 毒性； • 防止产品变成其他药物； • 禁止使用可能吸引儿童和青少年的酒精和甜味香料； • 要求制造商和进口商向政府机构披露水烟烟草的成分及释放物信息； • 要求制造商和进口商在政府机构登记。
	监督和监测。建议各国政府使用或加强现有的烟草监督和监测系统，以评估不同群体（包括不同性别和不同年龄）水烟使用的当前流行程度和未来演化。
	火灾风险评估。木炭的使用存在火灾隐患，对监管提出了挑战，应对其进行评估，缔约方应考虑建立用于火险评估目的的监测系统[1]。

11. 监管措施建议

TobReg 还提出了特别针对水烟的监管措施建议[179]。

WHO FCTC 条款	监管措施建议
第 6 条 a	依据 WHO FCTC 第 6 条，缔约方应对烟草制品实施税收措施，并限制或禁止免税烟草和水烟制品的进口和销售。
b	烟草税收的目的是通过提高成本来减少购买量从而降低需求量。因此，烟草税收实际上应该是很高的。如果水烟烟草只是按量（例如按千克计算）来征税，那么对消费者个人来说仍然相对便宜。缔约方应考虑按照个体消费量或更高的价格征税。
c	水烟本身及其部件和配件，也应纳税。
d	水烟、水烟烟草、部件和配件应禁止或限制免税销售。
第 8 条	水烟咖啡馆或水烟休息室不得像某些传统抽吸水烟的国家那样，豁免于室内清洁空气相关法规。应禁止在室内公共场所抽吸水烟，只允许在室外抽吸。不应允许在大型购物中心（例如室内的商场）内设置水烟场所。
第 9 条和第 10 条	水烟烟草和水烟烟气应按照与卷烟烟草同样严格的标准进行测试。相关法规应确保水烟烟草不得豁免于对成分或释放物的测试和管制。成分及释放物的测试结果应报告给政府相关部门。应制定有效措施，向公众传播关于抽吸水烟烟草的有害性和释放物信息。
第 11.1 条 a	**包装和标签上的健康声明。**根据 WHO FCTC 第 11 条，缔约方应禁止制造商和第三方对抽吸水烟烟草作出健康声明，并应禁止水烟健康或安全的虚假描述（例如"焦油含量 0% 或烟碱含量 0.05%"）。这也必须适用于配件，包括针对木炭的声明（"无味"，"无化学添加"，"100% 天然"）。即使是"不含烟草"或"草本"的水烟替代品也含有大量有害物质，其包装不得含有健康或安全声明。
b	**包装和标签上的健康警示。**健康警示应表明烟草使用的各种有害性，并应： • 经主管监管机构批准； • 按设定的时间间隔轮换（例如每隔 12 个月）； • 尺寸大，清晰，易懂，明显； • 覆盖面积不少于主显示区域的 30%（即不能隐藏在可能看不到的底部或侧面）

b	• 使用特定格式或包含图片的形式。
	警示标签必须置于水烟烟草包装上，包括水烟本身及其配件。仅标识水烟烟草是不够的，因为吸烟者可能看不到包装（如果他们在酒吧或咖啡馆抽吸）。鉴于水烟部件、木炭、过滤器和烟嘴可以单独售卖，所以警示标签应该贴在所有单独的包装上。
	管理方式应不仅限于在水烟上放置警示标签。除了功能性，水烟还有美观上的考虑，制造商和吸烟者可能会为了美观而抗拒或撕去标签。这应当是不被允许的。
	因为水烟警示标签的放置问题（在水烟本身及其配件上）面临新的挑战，所以在投放市场前进行警示标签放置的测试可能会有用，可以监测放置位置，从而找到成功的方案。
第 12 条 a	应实施关于抽吸水烟危害性的全面教育和公众认知计划。该计划应着重解决抽吸水烟比抽吸卷烟更安全或更健康的谬误。
b	应该广泛提供关于戒烟好处的教育和计划。
c	应为卫生工作者、社区工作者、社会工作者、媒体专业人员、教育工作者、决策者、管理人员和所有在烟草控制和卫生保健方面至关重要的人员提供抽吸水烟有害性的培训和认识。
第 13 条 a	任何形式的水烟广告、促销和赞助必须由相关政府机构监管。最容易做到这点的办法是确保将水烟毫无例外地纳入所有卷烟广告、促销和赞助的立法和监管范畴内。
b	监管措施必须适应水烟售卖的独特特征，即大多数广告、推广和销售都是通过互联网来进行。
c	缔约方对水烟的广告、促销和赞助的管制至少应做到：
	• 不能吸引非吸烟者或非烟碱使用者或者将他们作为销售目标，不管明示还是暗示；
	• 不能吸引未成年人（包括通过少儿节目未成年人出现的地点或场合，或者通过倡导性或暴力的漫画），不管明示还是暗示；
	• 鼓励戒烟，如果可能的话开通戒烟热线；
	• 不得含有健康、安全或医用声明；
	• 不得破坏任何烟草控制措施，包括不得推动水烟咖啡馆豁免于室内清洁空气政策；
	• 包含产品成分的真实信息，且不得歪曲相关风险的事实；
	• 不得将这些产品与赌博、酒精、非法药物或使用它们是不安全或不明智的活动或地点联系在一起；
	• 明确声称烟碱的致瘾性，以及这些产品就是在递送烟碱；
	• 禁止水烟具有正面影响的暗示。

d	为了积极地防止不恰当的市场行为，水烟广告、促销和赞助的所有授权形式必须在出版或传播之前获相关机构批准，之后对其进行监测以评估是否符合审批。
第 14 条	针对烟草依赖的戒断计划应包括对水烟抽吸依赖。应针对水烟抽吸有吸引力从而很难戒断的特点进行干预，这些特点包括： • 香味的吸引力； • 令人愉悦的气泡声； • 社会氛围或共用水烟的紧密联系。

12. 参考文献

[1] WHO Study Group on Tobacco Product Regulation (TobReg). Advisory note. Waterpipe tobacco smoking: health effects, research needs and recommended actions by regulators. Geneva: World Health Organization; 2005.

[2] Control and prevention of waterpipe tobacco products (document FCTC/COP/6/11). Conference of the Parties to the WHO Framework Convention on Tobacco Control, Sixth session, Moscow, Russian Federation, 13–18 October 2014. Geneva: World Health Organization; 2014.

[3] Goodman J. Tobacco in history: the cultures of dependence. London: Routledge; 1993.

[4] Benedict CA. Golden-silk smoke: a history of tobacco in China. Berkeley, California: University of California Press; 2011.

[5] Bhonsle RB, Murti PR, Gupta PC. Tobacco habits in India. In: Gupta PC, Hamner JE III, Murti PR, editors. Control of tobacco-related cancers and other diseases, proceedings of an international symposium. Bombay: Oxford University Press; 1992.

[6] Chattopadhyay A. Emperor Akbar as a healer and his eminent physicians. Bull Indian Inst History Med 2000;30:151-8.

[7] Maziak W, Eissenberg T, Ward KD. Patterns of waterpipe use and dependence: implications for intervention development. Pharmacol Biochem Behav 2005;80:173-9.

[8] Rastam S, Ward KD, Eissenberg T, Maziak W. Estimating the beginning of the waterpipe epidemic in Syria. BMC Public Health 2004;4:32.

[9] Maziak W, Taleb ZB, Bahelah R, Islam F, Jaber R, Auf R, et al. The global epidemiology of waterpipe smoking. Tob Control 2015;24(Suppl 1):i3-12.

[10] Martinasek MP, McDermott RJ, Martini L. Waterpipe (hookah) tobacco smoking among youth. Curr Probl Pediatr Adolesc Health Care 2011;41:34–57.

[11] Sutfin EL, Song EY, Reboussin BA, Wolfson M. What are young adults smoking in their hookahs? A latent class analysis of substances smoked. Addict Behav 2014;39:1191–6.

[12] Akl E, Ward KD, Bteddini D, Khaliel R, Alexander AC, Loutfi T, et al. The allure of the waterpipe: a narrative review of factors affecting the epidemic rise in waterpipe smoking among young persons globally. Tob Control 2015;24(Suppl 1):i13–21.

[13] Maziak W, Ward K, Soweid RAA, Eissenberg T. Tobacco smoking using a waterpipe: a reemerging strain in a global epidemic. Tob Control 2004;13:327–33.

[14] Maziak W, Nakkash R, Bahelah R, Husseini A, Fanous N, Eissenberg T. Tobacco in the Arab world: old and new epidemics amidst policy paralysis. Health Policy Plan 2013;29:784–94.

[15] Carroll MV, Chang J, Sidani JE, Barnett TE, Soule E, Balbach E, et al. Reigniting tobacco ritual: waterpipe tobacco smoking establishment culture in the United States. Nicotine Tob Res 2014;16:1549–58.

[16] Afifi R, Khalil J, Fouad F, Hammal F, Jarallah Y, Abu Farhat H, et al. Social norms and attitudes linked to waterpipe use in the Eastern Mediterranean Region. Soc Sci Med 2013;98:125–34.

[17] Tobacco policy trend alert. An emerging deadly trend: waterpipe tobacco use. Chicago, Illinois: American Lung Association; 2007 (http://www.lungusa2.org/ embargo/slati/ Trendalert_Waterpipes.pdf, accessed 5 July 2014).

[18] Nakkash RT, Khalil J, Afifi RA. The rise in narghile (shisha, hookah) waterpipe tobacco smoking: a qualitative study of perceptions of smokers and non smokers. BMC Public Health 2011;11:315.

[19] Sutfin E, McCoy TP, Reboussin BA, Wagoner KG, Spangler J, Wolfson M. Prevalence and correlates of waterpipe tobacco smoking by college students in North Carolina. Drug Alcohol Depend 2011;115:131–6.

[20] Salloum RG, Osman A, Maziak W, Thrasher JF. How popular is waterpipe tobacco smoking? Findings from Internet search queries. Tob Control. 2014 Jul 22. pii: tobaccocontrol-2014-051675. doi: 10.1136/tobaccocontrol-2014-051675.

[21] Primack BA, Rice KR, Shensa A, Carroll MV, DePenna EJ, Nakkash R, et al. US hookah tobacco smoking establishments advertised on the Internet. Am J Prev Med 2012;42:150-6.

[22] Carroll MV, Shensa A, Primack BA. A comparison of cigarette- and hookah-related videos on YouTube. Tob Control 2013;22:319-23.

[23] Brockman LN, Pumper MA, Christakis DA, Moreno MA. Hookah's new popularity among US college students: a pilot study of the characteristics of hookah smokers and their Facebook displays. BMJ Open 2012;2. pii: e001709.

[24] Salloum RG, Nakkash RT, Myers AE, Wood KA, Ribisl KM. Point-of-sale tobacco advertising in Beirut, Lebanon following a national advertising ban. BMC Public Health 2013;13:534.

[25] Bahelah R. Waterpipe tobacco labeling and packaging and World Health Organization Framework Convention on Tobacco Control (WHO FCTC): a call for action. Addiction 2014;109:333.

[26] Sepetdjian E, Shihadeh A, Saliba NA. Measurement of 16 polycyclic aromatic hydrocarbons in narghile waterpipe tobacco smoke. Food Chem Toxicol 2008;46:1582-90.

[27] Knishkowy B, Amitai Y. Water-pipe (narghile) smoking: an emerging health risk behavior. Pediatrics 2005;116:e113-9.

[28] Chaloupka FJ, Straif K, Leon ME. Effectiveness of tax and price policies in tobacco control. Tob Control 2011;20:235-8.

[29] Gilmore AB, Tavakoly B, Taylor G, Reed H. Understanding tobacco industry pricing strategy and whether it undermines tobacco tax policy: the example of the UK cigarette market. Addiction 2013;108:1317-26.

[30] El-Awa F, Warren C, Jones N. Changes in tobacco use among 13-15-year-olds between 1999 and 2007: findings from the Eastern Mediterranean Region. East

Med Health J 2010;16:266–73.

[31] Akl EA, Gunukula SK, Aleem S, Obeid R, Abou Jaoude P, Honeine R, et al. The prevalence of waterpipe tobacco smoking among the general and specific populations: a systematic review. BMC Public Health 2011;11:244.

[32] Maziak W. The waterpipe: time for action. Addiction 2008;103:1763–7.

[33] Maziak W. The global epidemic of waterpipe smoking. Addict Behav 2011;36:1–5.

[34] Morton J, Song Y, Fouad H, Awa FE, Abou El Naga R, et al. Cross country comparison of waterpipe use: nationally representative data from 13 low and middle-income countries from the Global Adult Tobacco Survey (GATS). Tob Control 2014;23:419–27.

[35] Attitudes of Europeans towards tobacco. Special Eurobarometer 385. Brussels: European Commission; 2012 (http://ec.europa.eu/health/tobacco/docs/eurobaro_attitudes_towards_ tobacco_2012_en.pdf).

[36] Smith-Simone S, Maziak W, Ward KD, Eissenberg T. Waterpipe tobacco smoking: knowledge, attitudes, beliefs, and behavior in two US samples. Nicotine Tob Res 2008;10:393–8.

[37] Maziak W, Ward KD, Eissenberg T. Factors related to frequency of narghile (waterpipe) use: the first insights on tobacco dependence in narghile users. Drug Alcohol Depend 2004;76:101–6.

[38] Warren CW, Lea V, Lee J, Jones NR, Asma S, McKenna M. Change in tobacco use among 13–15 year olds between 1999 and 2008: findings from the Global Youth Tobacco Survey. Global Health Promot 2009;16(Suppl):38–90.

[39] Rice VH, Weglicki LS, Templin T, Hammad A, Jamil H, Kulwicki A. Predictors of Arab American adolescent tobacco use. Merrill-Palmer Q J Dev Psychol 2006;52:327–42.

[40] Weglicki LS, Templin T, Hammad A, Jamil H, Abou-Mediene S, Farroukh M, et al. Tobacco use patterns among high school students: Do Arab American youth differ? Ethnicity Dis 2007; 17(Suppl 3): 22–4.

[41] Rice VH, Templin T, Hammad A, Weglicki L, Jamil H, Abou-Mediene S. Collab-

orative research of tobacco use and its predictors in Arab and non-Arab American 9th graders. Ethnicity Dis 2007;17(Suppl):19–21.

[42] El-Roueiheb Z, Tamim H, Kanj M, Jabbour S, Alayan I, Musharrafieh U. Cigarette and waterpipe smoking among Lebanese adolescents, a crosssectional study, 2003–2004. Nicotine Tob Res 2008;10:309–14.

[43] Primack BA, Sidani J, Agarwal AA, Shadel WG, Donny EC, Eissenberg TE. Prevalence of and associations with waterpipe tobacco smoking among US university students. Ann Behav Med 2008;36:81–6.

[44] Zoughaib SS, Adib SM, Jabbour J. Prevalence and determinants of water pipe or narghile use among students in Beirut's southern suburbs. J Med Liban 2004;52:142–8.

[45] Tamim H, Al-Sahab B, Akkary G, Ghanem M, Tamim N, El Roueiheb Z, et al. Cigarette and nargileh smoking practices among school students in Beirut, Lebanon. Am J Health Behav 2007;31:56–63.

[46] Taha AZA. Prevalence of risk-taking behaviors. Bahrain Med Bull 2007;29:1–10.

[47] Jackson D, Aveyard P. Waterpipe smoking in students: prevalence, risk factors, symptoms of addiction, and smoke intake. Evidence from one British university. BMC Public Health 2008;8:174.

[48] Jawaid A, Zafar AM, Rehman TU, Nazir MR, Ghafoor ZA, Afzal O, et al. Knowledge, attitudes and practice of university students regarding waterpipe smoking in Pakistan. Int J Tuberc Lung Dis 2008;12:1077–84.

[49] Senkubuge F, Ayo-Yusuf OA, Louwagie GM, Okuyemi KS. Water pipe and smokeless tobacco use among medical students in South Africa. Nicotine Tob Res 2012;14:755–760.

[50] Combrink A, Irwin N, Laudin G, Naidoo K, Plagerson S, Mathee A. High prevalence of hookah smoking among secondary school students in a disadvantaged community in Johannesburg. S Afr Med J 2010;100:297–9.

[51] Daniels K, Roman N. A descriptive study of the perceptions and behaviors of waterpipe use by university students in the Western Cape, South Africa. Tob In-

duced Dis 2013;11:4.

[52] Global adult tobacco survey: Nigeria country report 2012. Brazzaville: World Health Organization Regional Office for Africa.

[53] Khattab A, Javaid A, Iraqi G, Alzaabi A, Ben Kheder A, Koniski ML, et al. Smoking habits in the Middle East and North Africa: results of the BREATHE study. Respir Med 2012;106(Suppl 2):S16–24.

[54] Czoli CD, Leatherdale ST, Rynard V. Bidi and hookah use among Canadian youth: findings from the 2010 Canadian Youth Smoking Survey. Prev Chronic Dis 2013;10:120290.

[55] Agaku IT, King BA, Husten CG, Bunnell R, Ambrose BK, Hu SS, et al. Tobacco product use among adults—United States, 2012–2013. Morbid Mortal Wkly Rep 2014;63:542–7.

[56] Amrock SM, Gordon T, Zelikoff JT, Weitzman M. Hookah use among adolescents in the United States: results of a national survey. Nicotine Tob Res 2014;16:231–7.

[57] Palamar JJ, Zhou S, Sherman S, Weitzman M. Hookah use among US high school seniors. Pediatrics 2014;134:1–8.

[58] Global Adult Tobacco Survey: Argentina 2012. Buenos Aires: Government of Argentina, 2013.

[59] Shihadeh A, Azar S, Antonios C, Haddad A. Towards a topographical model of narghile water-pipe café smoking: a pilot study in a high socioeconomic status neighborhood of Beirut, Lebanon. Biochem Pharmacol Behav 2004;79:75–82.

[60] Warren C, Jones N, Eriksen M, Asma S. Patterns of global tobacco use in young people and implications for future chronic disease burden in adults. Lancet 2006;367:749–53.

[61] Mzayek F, Khader Y, Eissenberg T, Al Ali R, Ward KD, Maziak W. Patterns of water-pipe and cigarette smoking initiation in schoolchildren: Irbid Longitudinal Smoking Study. Nicotine Tob Res 2012;14:448–54.

[62] Moh'd Al-Mulla A, Abdou Helmy S, Al-Lawati J, Al Nasser S, Ali Abdel Rahman S, Almutawa A, et al. Prevalence of tobacco use among students aged 13–15

years in Health Ministers' Council/Gulf Cooperation Council Member States, 2001–2004. J School Health 2008;78:337–43.

[63] Global Adult Tobacco Survey: Egypt country report 2009. Cairo: World Health Organization Regional Office for the Eastern Mediterranean.

[64] Global Adult Tobacco Survey: GATS Qatar 2013 fact sheet. Doha: Government of Qatar.

[65] Sorina I, editor. Global Adult Tobacco Survey—Romania 2011. Cluj-Napoca: Eikon, 2012.

[66] Jawad M, Abass J, Hariri A, Rajasooriar KG, Salmasi H, Millett C, et al. Water-pipe smoking prevalence and attitudes amongst medical students in London. Int J Tuberc Lung Dis 2013;17:137–40.

[67] Jawad M, Wilson A, Lee LT, Jawad S, Hamilton FL, Millet C. Prevalence and pre-dictors of water pipe and cigarette smoking among secondary school students in London. Nicotine Tob Res 2013;15:2069–75.

[68] Slama K, David-Tchouda S, Plassart J. Tobacco consumption among young adults in the two French departments of Savoie in 2008. Rev Epidémiol Santé Publique 2009;57:299–304.

[69] Pärna K, Usin J, Ringmets I. Cigarette and waterpipe smoking among adolescents in Estonia: HBSC survey results, 1994–2006. BMC Public Health 2008;8:392.

[70] Varsano S, Ganz I, Eldor N, Garenkin M. Water-pipe tobacco smoking among school children in Israel: frequencies, habits, and attitudes. Harefuah 2003;142:736–41.

[71] Korn L. The nargila smoking phenomenon among teen-agers in Israel: a socio-logical analysis. PhD thesis. Ramat-Gan: Bar-Ilan University, Department of Sociology and Anthropology; 2005.

[72] Korn L, Harel-Fisch Y, Amitai G. Social and behavioral determinants of nargila (water-pipe) smoking among Israeli youth: findings from the 2002 HBSC sur-vey. J Subst Use 2008;13:225–38.

[73] Harel Y, Molcho M, Tillinger E. Youth in Israel. Health, well-being and risk

behaviors. Summary of findings from the third national study (2002) and trend analysis (1994–2002). Ramat-Gan: Bar-Ilan University, Department of Sociology and Anthropology; 2003.

[74] Global Adult Tobacco Survey: Indonesia Report 2011. New Delhi: World Health Organization Regional Office for South East Asia.

[75] GATS India Report 2009–2010. New Delhi: Ministry of Health and Family Welfare, Government of India; 2011.

[76] She J, Yang P, Wang Y, Qin X, Fan J, Wang Y, et al. Chinese waterpipe smoking and the risk of chronic obstructive pulmonary disease. Chest 2014;146:924–31.

[77] Report of the Global Adult Tobacco Survey (GATS) Malaysia, 2011. Kuala Lumpur: Institute for Public Health, Ministry of Health Malaysia; 2012.

[78] Personal habits and indoor combustions. IARC Monographs on the Carcinogenic Risk of Chemicals to Humans, Vol. 100E. Lyon: International Agency for Research on Cancer; 2012.

[79] Kassem NOF, Kassem NO, Jackson SR, Liles S, Daffa RM, Zarth AT, et al. Benzene uptake in hookah smokers and non-smokers attending hookah social events: regulatory implications. Cancer Epidemiol Biomarkers Prev 2014;146:924–31.

[80] Saleh R, Shihadeh A. Elevated toxicant yields with narghile waterpipes smoked using a plastic hose. Food Chem Toxicol 2008;46:1461–6.

[81] Apsley A, Galea KS, Sánchez Jiménez A, Semple S, Wareing H, Tongeren MV. Assessment of polycyclic aromatic hydrocarbons, carbon monoxide, nicotine, metal contents and particle size distribution of mainstream shisha smoke. J Environ Health Res 2011;11:93.

[82] Jenkins R, Guerin M, Tomkins B. The chemistry of environmental tobacco smoke. Boca Raton, Florida: Lewis Publishers; 2000.

[83] Monzer B, Sepetdjian E, Saliba N, Shihadeh A. Charcoal emissions as a source of CO and carcinogenic PAH in mainstream narghile waterpipe smoke. Food Chem Toxicol 2008; 46:2991–5.

[84] Schubert J, Hahn J, Dettbarn G, Seidel A, Luch A, Schulz TG. Mainstream

smoke of the waterpipe: Does this environmental matrix reveal as significant source of toxic compounds? Toxicol Lett 2001;205:279–84.

[85] Shihadeh A. Investigation of mainstream smoke aerosol of the argileh water pipe. Food Chem Toxicol 2003;41:143–52.

[86] Bentur L, Hellou E, Goldbart A, Pillar G, Monovich E, Salameh M, et al. Laboratory and clinical acute effects of active and passive indoor group water-pipe (narghile) smoking. Chest 2014;145:803–9.

[87] St Helen G, Benowitz NL, Dains KM, Havel C, Peng M, Jacob P 3rd. Nicotine and carcinogen exposure after water pipe smoking in hookah bars. Cancer Epidemiol Biomarkers Prev 2014;23:1055–66.

[88] Cobb CO, Sahmarani K, Eissenberg T, Shihadeh A. Acute toxicant exposure and cardiac autonomic dysfunction from smoking a single narghile waterpipe with tobacco and with a "healthy" tobacco-free alternative. Toxicol Lett 2012;215:70–5.

[89] Al Ali R, Rastam S, Ibrahim I, Bazzi A, Fayad S, Shihadeh AL, et al. A comparative study of systemic carcinogen exposure in waterpipe smokers, cigarette smokers and non-smokers. Tob Control 2015;24:125–7.

[90] Jacob P, Raddaha AHA, Dempsey D, Havel C, Peng M, Yu L, et al. Nicotine, carbon monoxide, and carcinogen exposure after a single use of a water pipe. Cancer Epidemiol Biomarkers Prev 2011;20:2345–53.

[91] Jacob P, Raddaha AHA, Dempsey D, Havel C, Peng M, Yu L, et al. Comparison of nicotine and carcinogen exposure with water pipe and cigarette smoking. Cancer Epidemiol Biomarkers Prev 2013;22:765–72.

[92] El Zaatari ZM, Chami HA, Zaatari, GS. Health effects associated with waterpipe smoking. Tob Control 2015;24(Suppl 1):i31–43.

[93] Lim BL, Lim GH, Seow E. Case of carbon monoxide poisoning after smoking shisha. Int J Emerg Med 2009;2:121–2.

[94] La Fauci G, Weiser G, Steiner IP, Shavit I. Carbon monoxide poisoning in narghile (water pipe) tobacco smokers. Can J Emerg Med 2012;14:57–9.

[95] Alomari MA, Khabour OF, Alzoubi KH, Shqair DM, Eissenberg T. Central and

peripheral cardiovascular changes immediately after waterpipe smoking. Inhal Toxicol 2014;26:579–87.

[96] Hakim F, Hellou E, Goldbart A, Katz R, Bentur Y, Bentur L. The acute effects of water-pipe smoking on the cardiorespiratory system. Chest 2011;139:775–81.

[97] Eissenberg T, Shihadeh A. Waterpipe tobacco and cigarette smoking: direct comparison of toxicant exposure. Am J Prev Med 2009;37:518–23.

[98] Al-Kubati M, Al-Kubati AS, Al'Absi M, Fišer B. The short-term effect of water-pipe smoking on the baroreflex control of heart rate in normotensives. Autonomic Neurosci 2006;126:146–9.

[99] Hawari FI, Obeidat NA, Ayub H, Ghonimat I, Eissenberg T, Dawahrah S, et al. The acute effects of waterpipe smoking on lung function and exercise capacity in a pilot study of healthy participants. Inhal Toxicol 2013;25:492–7.

[100] Markowicz P, Löndahl J, Wierzbicka A, Suleiman R, Shihadeh A, Larsson L. A study on particles and some microbial markers in waterpipe tobacco smoke. Sci Total Environ 2014;499:107–13.

[101] Fromme H, Dietrich S, Heitmann D, Dressel H, Diemer J, Schulz T, et al. Indoor air contamination during a waterpipe (narghile) smoking session. Food Chem Toxicol 2009;47:1636–41.

[102] Cobb CO, Vansickel AR, Blank MD, Jentink K, Travers MJ, Eissenberg T. Indoor air quality in Virginia waterpipe cafes. Tob Control 2013;22:338–43.

[103] Hammal F, Chappell A, Wild TC, Kindzierski W, Shihadeh A, Vanderhoek A, et al. "Herbal" but potentially hazardous: an analysis of the constituents and smoke emissions of tobaccofree waterpipe products and the air quality in the cafés where they are served. Tob Control 2015;24:290–7.

[104] Maziak W, Ibrahim I, Rastam S, Ward KD, Eissenberg T. Waterpipe-associated particulate matter emissions. Nicotine Tob Res 2008;10:519–23.

[105] Daher N, Saleh R, Jaroudi E, Sheheitli H, Badr T, Sepetdijan E, et al. Comparison of carcinogen, carbon monoxide, and ultrafine particle emissions from narghile waterpipe and cigarette smoking: sidestream smoke measurements and as-

sessment of second-hand smoke emission factors. Atmos Environ 2010;44:8–14.

[106] Akl EA, Gaddam S, Gunukula SK, Honeine R, Jaoude PA, Irani J. The effects of waterpipe tobacco smoking on health outcomes: a systematic review. Int J Epidemiol 2010;39:834–57.

[107] Dangi J, Kinnunen TH, Zavras AI. Challenges in global improvement of oral cancer outcomes: findings from rural northern India. Tob Induced Dis 2012;10:5.

[108] Ali AA, Ali AA. Histopathologic changes in oral mucosa of Yemenis addicted to water-pipe and cigarette smoking in addition to takhzeen al-qat. Oral Surg Oral Med Oral Pathol Oral Radiol Endod 2007;103:e55–9.

[109] Nasrollahzadeh D, Kamangar F, Aghcheli K, Sotoudeh M, Islami F, Abnet CC, et al. Opium, tobacco, and alcohol use in relation to oesophageal squamous cell carcinoma in a high-risk area of Iran. Br J Cancer 2008;98:1857–63.

[110] Dar NA, Bhat GA, Shah IA, Iqbal B, Makhdoomi MA, Nisar I, et al. Hookah smoking, nass chewing, and oesophageal squamous cell carcinoma in Kashmir, India. Br J Cancer 2012;107:1618–23.

[111] Malik MA, Upadhyay R, Mittal RD, Zargar SA, Mittal B. Association of xenobiotic metabolizing enzymes genetic polymorphisms with esophageal cancer in Kashmir Valley and influence of environmental factors. Nutr Cancer 2010;62:734–42.

[112] Qiao YL, Taylor PR, Yao SX, Schatzkin A, Mao BL, Lubin J, et al. Relation of radon exposure and tobacco use to lung cancer among tin miners in Yunnan Province, China. Am J Ind Med 1989;16:511–21.

[113] Gupta D, Boffetta P, Gaborieau V, Jindal SK. Risk factors of lung cancer in Chandigarh, India. Indian J Med Res 2001;113:142–50.

[114] Lubin JH, Qiao YL, Taylor PR, Yao SX, Schatzkin A, Mao BL, et al. Quantitative evaluation of the radon and lung cancer association in a case control study of Chinese tin miners. Cancer Res 1990;50:174–80.

[115] Lubin JH, Li JY, Xuan XZ, Cai SK, Luo QS, Yang LF, et al. Risk of lung cancer among cigarette and pipe smokers in southern China. Int J Cancer 1992;51:390–5.

[116] Hsairi M, Achour N, Zouari B. Facteurs etiologiques du cancer bronchique

primitif en Tunisie. [Etiological factors for primary lung cancer in Tunisia.] Tunisie Med 1993;71:265–8.

[117] Hazelton WD, Luebeck EG, Heidenreich WF, Moolgavkar SH. Analysis of a historical cohort of Chinese tin miners with arsenic, radon, cigarette smoke, and pipe smoke exposures using the biologically based two-stage clonal expansion model. Radiat Res 2001;156:78–94.

[118] Sadjadi A, Derakhshan MH, Yazdanbod A, Boreiri M, Persaeian M, Babaei M, et al. Neglected role of hookah and opium in gastric carcinogenesis: a cohort study on risk factors and attributable fractions. Int J Cancer 2014;134:181–8.

[119] Shakeri R, Malekzadeh R, Etemadi A, Nasrollahzadeh D, Aghcheli K, Sotoudeh M, et al. Opium: an emerging risk factor for gastric adenocarcinoma. Int J Cancer 2013;133:455–61.

[120] Bedwani R, El-Khwsky F, Renganathan E, Braga C, Abu Seif HH, Abul Azm T, et al. Epidemiology of bladder cancer in Alexandria, Egypt: tobacco smoking. Int J Cancer 1997;73:64–7.

[121] Zheng YL, Amr S, Saleh DA, Dash C, Ezzat S, Mikhail NN, et al. Urinary bladder cancer risk factors in Egypt: a multicenter case-control study. Cancer Epidemiol Biomarkers Prev 2012;21:537–46.

[122] Mohammad Y, Shaaban R, Abou Al-Zahab B, Khaltaev N, Bousquet J, Dubaybo B. Impact of active and passive smoking as risk factors for asthma and COPD in women presenting to primary care in Syria: first report by the WHO-GARD survey group. Int J Chron Obstruct Pulmon Dis 2013;8: 473–82.

[123] Waked M, Khayat G, Salameh P. Chronic obstructive pulmonary disease prevalence in Lebanon: a cross-sectional descriptive study. Clin Epidemiol 2011;3:315–23.

[124] Tageldin MA, Nafti S, Khan JA, Nejjari C, Beji M, Mahboub B, et al. Distribution of COPDrelated symptoms in the Middle East and North Africa: results of the BREATHE study. Respir Med 2012;106(Suppl 2):S25–32.

[125] Waked M, Salameh P, Aoun Z. Water-pipe (narguile) smokers in Lebanon: a pi-

lot study. East Med Health J 2009;15: 432–42.

[126] Salameh P, Waked M, Khoury F, Akiki Z, Nasser Z, Abou Abass L, et al. Water-pipe smoking and dependence are associated with chronic bronchitis: a case-control study in Lebanon. East Med Health J 2012;18:996–1004.

[127] Salameh P, Waked M, Khayat G, Dramaix M. Waterpipe smoking and dependence are associated with chronic obstructive pulmonary disease: a case–control study. Open Epidemiol J 2012;5:36–44.

[128] Sekine Y, Katsura H, Koh E, Hiroshima K, Fujisawa T. Early detection of COPD is important for lung cancer surveillance. Eur Respir J 2012;39: 1230–40.

[129] Sibai AM, Tohme RA, Almedawar MM, Itani T, Yassine SI, Nohra EA, et al. Lifetime cumulative exposure to waterpipe smoking is associated with coronary artery disease. Atherosclerosis 2014;234:454–60.

[130] Wu F, Chen Y, Parvez F, Segers S, Argos M, Islam T, et al. A prospective study of tobacco smoking and mortality in Bangladesh. PLoS One 2013;8:e58516.

[131] Islami F, Pourshams A, Vednathan R, Poustchi H, Kamangar F, Golozar A, et al. Smoking water-pipe, chewing nass and prevalence of heart disease: a cross-sectional analysis of baseline data from the Golestan Cohort Study, Iran. Heart 2013;99:272–8.

[132] Selim GM, Fouad H, Ezzat S. Impact of shisha smoking on the extent of coronary artery disease in patients referred for coronary angiography. Anadolu Kardiyol Derg 2013;13:647–54.

[133] El-Sadawy M, Ragab H, El-Toukhy H, El Latif El Mor A, Mangoud AM, Eissa MH, et al. Hepatitis C virus infection at Sharkia Governorate, Egypt: seroprevalence and associated risk factors. J Egypt Soc Parasitol 2004;34(1 Suppl):367–84.

[134] Habib M, Mohamed MK, Abdel-Aziz F, Magder LS, Abdel-Hamid M, Gamil F, et al. Hepatitis C virus infection in a community in the Nile Delta: risk factors for seropositivity. Hepatology 2001;33:248–53.

[135] Medhat A, Shehata M, Magder LS, Mikhail N, Abdel-Baki M, Nafeh M, et al. Hepatitis C in a community in Upper Egypt: risk factors for infection. Am J

Trop Med Hyg 2002;66:633–8.

[136] Steentoft J, Wittendorf J, Andersen JR. Tuberkulose og vandpibesmitte [Tuberculosis and water pipes as source of infection]. Ugeskr Laeg 2006;168:904–7.

[137] Munckhof WJ, Konstaninos A, Wamsley M, Mortlock M, Gilpin C. A cluster of tuberculosis associated with use of a marijuana water pipe. Int J Tuberc Lung Dis 2003:7:860–5.

[138] Salamé J, Salameh P, Khayat G, Waked M. Cigarette and waterpipe smoking decrease respiratory quality of life in adults: results from a national cross-sectional study. Pulm Med 2012;2012:868294.

[139] Tavafian SS, Aghamolaei T, Zare S. Water pipe smoking and health-related quality of life: a population-based study. Arch Iran Med 2009;12:232–7.

[140] Tamim H, Yunis KA, Chemaitelly H, Alameh M, Nassar AH, National Collaborative Perinatal Neonatal Network Beirut, Lebanon. Effect of narghile and cigarette smoking on newborn birthweight. B J Obst Gynaecol 2008;115:91–7.

[141] Nuwayhid IA, Yamout B, Azar G, Kambris MA. Narghile (hubble-bubble) smoking, low birth weight, and other pregnancy outcomes. Am J Epidemiol 1998;148:375–83.

[142] Aghamolaei T, Eftekhar H, Zare S. Risk factors associated with intrauterine growth retardation (IUGR) in Bandar Abbas. J Med Sci 2007;7:665–9.

[143] Al-Belasy FA, Al-Belasy FA. The relationship of "shisha" (water pipe) smoking to postextraction dry socket. J Oral Maxillofac Surg 2004;62:10–4.

[144] Natto S, Baljoon M, Bergstrom J. Tobacco smoking and periodontal bone height in a Saudi Arabian population. J Clin Periodontol 2005;32:1000–6.

[145] Natto S, Baljoon M, Abanmy A, Bergstrom J. Tobacco smoking and gingival health in a Saudi Arabian population. Oral Health Prev Dent 2004;2:351–7.

[146] Natto S, Baljoon M, Bergstrom J. Tobacco smoking and periodontal health in a Saudi Arabian population. J Periodontol 2005;76:1919–26.

[147] Baljoon M, Natto S, Abanmy A, Bergström J. Smoking and vertical bone defects in a Saudi Arabian population. Oral Health Prev Dent 2005;3:173–82.

[148] Tamim H, Musharrafieh U, El Roueiheb Z, Yunis K, Almawi WY. Exposure of children to environmental tobacco smoke (ETS) and its association with respiratory ailments. J Asthma 2003;40:571–6.

[149] Islami F, Nasseri-Moghaddam S, Pourshams A, Poustchi H, Semnani S, et al. Determinants of gastroesophageal reflux disease, including hookah smoking and opium use—a cross-sectional analysis of 50,000 individuals. PLoS One 2014;9:e89256.

[150] Primack BA, Land SR, Fan J, Kim KH, Rosen D. Associations of mental health problems with waterpipe tobacco and cigarette smoking among college students. Subst Use Misuse 2013;48:211–9.

[151] Maziak W, Ward KD, Eissenberg T. Interventions for waterpipe smoking cessation. Cochrane Database Syst Rev 2011;6:CD005549.

[152] Macaron C, Macaron Z, Maalouf MT, Macaron N, Moore A. Urinary cotinine in narguila or chicha tobacco smokers. J Med Liban 1997;45:19–20.

[153] Maziak W, Rastam S, Shihadeh AL, Bazzi A, Ibrahim I, Zaatari GS, et al. Nicotine exposure in daily waterpipe smokers and its relation to puff topography. Addict Behav 2011;36:397–9.

[154] Eissenberg T, Shihadeh A. Waterpipe tobacco and cigarette smoking: direct comparison of toxicant exposure. Am J Prev Med 2009;37:518–23.

[155] Ward KD, Hammal F, VanderWeg MW, Eissenberg, Asfar T, Rastam S, et al. Are waterpipe users interested in quitting? Nicotine Tob Res 2005;7:149–56.

[156] Maziak W, Rastam S, Ward KD, Shihadeh AL, Eissenberg T. CO exposure, puff topography, and subjective effects in waterpipe tobacco smokers. Nicotine Tob Res 2009;11:806–11.

[157] Hammal F, Mock J, Ward KD, Eissenberg T, Maziak W. A pleasure among friends: how narghile (waterpipe) smoking differs from cigarette smoking in Syria. Tob Control 2008;17:e3.

[158] Maynard OM, Gage SH, Munafò MR. Are waterpipe users tobacco-dependent? Addiction 2013;108:1886–7.

[159] Maziak W, Ward KD, Afifi Soweid RA, Eissenberg T. Standardizing question-naire items for the assessment of waterpipe tobacco use in epidemiological studies. Public Health 2005;119:400–4.

[160] Salameh P, Waked M, Aoun Z. Waterpipe smoking: construction and validation of the Lebanon Waterpipe Dependence Scale (LWDS-11). Nicotine Tob Res 2008;10:149–58.

[161] Primack BA, Khabour OF, Alzoubi KH, Switzer GE, Shensa A, Carroll MV, et al. The LWDS-10J: reliability and validity of the Lebanon Waterpipe Dependence Scale among university students in Jordan. Nicotine Tob Res 2014;16:915–22.

[162] Aboaziza E, Eissenberg T. Waterpipe tobacco smoking: what is the evidence that it supports nicotine/tobacco dependence? Tob Control 2014;24(Suppl 1):i144–53.

[163] Salameh P, Khayat G, Waked M. Lower prevalence of cigarette and waterpipe smoking, but a higher risk of waterpipe dependence in Lebanese adult women than in men. Women Health 2012;52:135–50.

[164] Cobb C, Ward KD, Maziak W, Shihadeh AL, Eissenberg T. Waterpipe tobacco smoking: an emerging health crisis in the United States. Am J Health Behav 2010;34:275–85.

[165] Asfar T, VanderWeg MW, Maziak W, Hammal F, Eissenberg T, Ward KD. Outcomes and adherence in Syria's first smoking cessation trial. Am J Health Behav 2008;32:146–56.

[166] Rastam S, Eissenberg T, Ibrahim I, Ward KD, Khalil R, Maziak W. Comparative analysis of waterpipe and cigarette suppression of abstinence and craving symptoms. Addict Behav 2011;36:555–9.

[167] Jaber R, Madhivanan P, Veledar E, Khader Y, Mzayek F, Maziak W. Waterpipe a gateway to cigarette smoking among adolescents in Irbid, Jordan: a longitudinal study. Int J Tuberc Lung Dis 2015;19:481–7.

[168] Soneji S, Sargent JD, Tanski SE, Primack BA. Associations between initial water pipe tobacco smoking and snus use and subsequent cigarette smoking: results

from a longitudinal study of US adolescents and young adults. JAMA Pediatr 2015;169:129–36.

[169] Shihadeh AL, Eissenberg TE. Significance of smoking machine toxicant yields to blood-level exposure in water pipe tobacco smokers. Cancer Epidemiol Biomarkers Prev 2011;20:2457–60.

[170] Zyoud SH, Al-Jabi SW, Sweileh WM. Bibliometric analysis of scientific publications on waterpipe (narghile, shisha, hookah) tobacco smoking during the period 2003–2012. Tob Induced Dis 2014;12:7.

[171] Pepper JK, Eissenberg T. Waterpipes and electronic cigarettes: increasing prevalence and expanding science. Chem Res Toxicol 2014;27:1336–43.

[172] Jawad M, McEwen MN, Shahab L. To what extent should waterpipe tobacco smoking become a public health priority? Addiction 2013;108:1873–84.

[173] WHO Tobacco Laboratory Network. Standard operating procedure for determination of nicotine in cigarette tobacco filler. WHO Tobacco Laboratory Network (TobLabNet) official method. Standard operating procedure 04. Geneva: World Health Organization; 2014.

[174] WHO Tobacco Laboratory Network. Standard operating procedure for determination of tobacco-specific nitrosamines in mainstream cigarette smoke under ISO and intense smoking conditions. WHO Tobacco Laboratory Network (TobLabNet) official method. Standard operating procedure 03. Geneva: World Health Organization; 2014.

[175] WHO Tobacco Laboratory Network. Standard operating procedure for determination of benzo[a]pyrene in mainstream cigarette smoke under ISO and intense smoking conditions. WHO Tobacco Laboratory Network (TobLabNet) official method. Standard operating procedure 05. Geneva: World Health Organization; 2015.

[176] Further development of the partial guidelines for implementation of Articles 9 and 10 of the WHO FCTC (Decision FCTC/COP6(12)). Conference of the Parties to the WHO Framework Convention on Tobacco Control, Sixth session,

Moscow, Russian Federation, 13–18 October 2014. Geneva: World Health Organization; 2014.

[177] Shihadeh A, Schubert J, Klaiany J, El Sabban M, Luch A, Saliba NA. Toxicant content, physical properties and biological activity of waterpipe tobacco smoke and its tobacco-free alternatives. Tob Control 2014;24:e72–80.

[178] Khabour O, Alzoubi KH, Bani-Ahmad M, Dodin A, Eissenberg T, Shihadeh A. Acute exposure to waterpipe tobacco smoke induces changes in the oxidative and inflammatory markers in mouse lung. Inhal Toxicol 2012; 24:667–75.

[179] Control and prevention of waterpipe tobacco products (Decision FCTC/COP6(10)). Conference of the Parties to the WHO Framework Convention on Tobacco Control, Sixth session, Moscow, Russian Federation, 13–18 October 2014. Geneva: World Health Organization; 2014.

WHO Study Group on Tobacco Product Regulation

Members

Dr D. L. Ashley, Director, Office of Science, Center for Tobacco Products, Food and Drug Administration, Rockville, Maryland, United States of America

Professor O. A. Ayo-Yusuf, Dean, School of Oral Health Sciences, Sefako Makgatho Health Sciences University, Pretoria, South Africa

Professor A. R. Boobis, Centre for Pharmacology and Therapeutics, Department of Medicine, Imperial College, London; Director, Public Health England Toxicology Unit, Imperial College London, United Kingdom

Dr Vera Luiza da Costa e Silva, Independent Consultant, Senior Public Health Specialist, Rio de Janeiro, Brazil

Dr M. V. Djordjevic, Program Director/Project Officer, Tobacco Control Research Branch, Behavioral Research Program, Division of Cancer Control and Population Sciences, National Cancer Institute, Bethesda, Maryland, United States of America

Dr N. Gray, Honorary Senior Associate, Cancer Council Victoria, Melbourne, Australia[†]

Dr P. Gupta, Director, Healis Sekhsaria Institute for Public Health, Mumbai, India

Dr S. K. Hammond, Professor of Environmental Health Sciences, School of Public Health, University of California, Berkeley, California, United States of America

Dr D. Hatsukami, Professor of Psychiatry, University of Minnesota, Minneapolis, Minnesota, United States of America

Dr A. Opperhuizen, Director, Office for Risk Assessment and Research, Utrecht, The Netherlands

Dr G. Zaatari (Chair), Professor and Chairman, Department of Pathology and Laboratory Medicine, American University of Beirut, Beirut, Lebanon

Contributors

Dr E. Akl, Associate Professor of Medicine, Department of Internal Medicine, American University of Beirut, Lebanon

Dr T. Eissenberg, Professor of Psychology and Co-Director, Center for the Study of Tobacco Products, Virginia Commonwealth University, Richmond, Virginia, United States of America

Dr W. Maziak, Professor and Chair, Department of Epidemiology, Florida International University; Director, Syrian Center for Tobacco Studies, Miami, Florida, United States of America

Dr P. Mehrotra, Senior Programme Officer, Population Council, New Delhi, India

Mr J. Morton, Senior Survey Methodologist, Global Tobacco Control Branch, Office on Smoking and Health, Centers for Disease Control and Prevention, Atlanta, Georgia, United States of America

Dr A. Shihadeh, Professor of Mechanical Engineering, Faculty of Engineering and Architecture, American University of Beirut, Beirut, Lebanon

WHO Secretariat

(Tobacco Free Initiative, Prevention of Noncommunicable Diseases, Geneva, Switzerland)

Ms M. Aryee-Quansah, Administrative Assistant

Dr A. Peruga, Programme Manager

Ms G. Vestal, Technical Officer (Legal)

1. Preface

Tobacco product regulation, which involves regulating the contents and emissions of tobacco products by testing, mandating the disclosure of the test results and regulating the packaging and labelling of tobacco products, is one of the pillars of any comprehensive tobacco control programme. The WHO Framework Convention on Tobacco Control (WHO FCTC), a binding international treaty, acknowledges the importance of tobacco product regulation in Articles 9, 10 and 11, and Parties to the Convention are bound by the provisions of those articles.

A WHO scientific advisory group on tobacco product regulation was established in 2000 to fill the gaps in knowledge that existed at the time. The scientific information provided by that group served as a basis for the negotiations and the subsequent consensus reached on the language of those three articles of the Convention.

In November 2003, in recognition of the critical importance of regulating tobacco products, the WHO Director-General formalized the ad hoc Scientific Advisory Committee on Tobacco Product Regulation by changing its status to that of a study group, which became the WHO Study Group on Tobacco Product Regulation (TobReg). The Group is composed of national and international scientific experts on product regulation, treatment of tobacco dependence and the laboratory analysis of tobacco ingredients and emissions. Its work is based on scientific evidence from the latest research on tobacco product issues. It makes recommendations and proposes testing for filling regulatory gaps in tobacco control. As a formalized entity of WHO, TobReg reports to the WHO Executive Board through the Director-General to draw Member States' attention to the Organization's efforts in tobacco product regulation.

TobReg prepared the first edition of the advisory note *Waterpipe tobacco smoking: health effects, research needs and recommended actions by regulators (1)* in response to requests from Member States in which the population is particularly exposed to this form of tobacco use and in accordance with the priorities of the WHO Tobacco Free Initiative and the provisions of the WHO FCTC concerning tobacco product regulation. TobReg approved and adopted the advisory note at its second meeting, held in Rio de Janeiro, Brazil, in 2005. Since then, new information has become available, and scientific research has addressed some of the gaps identified at the time of the first edition. Moreover, the First International Conference on Waterpipe Tobacco Smoking, held in Abu Dhabi in October 2013, addressed the state of knowledge on this subject; this was followed by a second conference, on the theme "Waterpipe smoking research: a collision of two epidemics of waterpipe and cigarettes", held in Doha, Qatar, in October 2014. The participants at both conferences called on WHO to update the 2005 advisory note and to consider other actions to support Member States and Parties to the WHO FCTC in preventing and controlling waterpipe use and other forms of exposure to tobacco. In addition, in March 2014, several TobReg members and regional and international waterpipe experts attended a workshop held at the WHO Regional Office for the Eastern Mediterranean in Cairo, Egypt, where they discussed the scientific evidence, challenges, gaps and regulatory policy issues and agreed to write this second edition of the advisory note.

WHO commissioned the six contributors listed in the acknowledgements to draft the sections that form the backbone of this report. Further, WHO was requested by the Conference of the Parties to the WHO FCTC at its sixth session, in October 2014 in Moscow, Russian Federation, to prepare a report on the toxic contents and emissions of waterpipe tobacco products and also a report on policy options and best practices in the control of use of waterpipe tobacco products, to be submitted to the seventh session of the Conference of the Parties to the WHO FCTC. WHO therefore invited TobReg to issue a second edition of the advisory note on the health effects, research needs and recommended actions for regulators with regard to waterpipe tobacco smoking. Section 7 addresses the health effects of the toxic contents and emissions of waterpipes, section 10 recommends policy, and section 11 gives recommendations for regulators. TobReg is pleased to present this second edition of the advisory note on waterpipe smoking.

TobReg members serve without remuneration in their personal capacities rather than as representatives of governments or other bodies; their views do not necessarily reflect the decisions or stated policies of WHO. The members' names are provided in this report.

2. Acknowledgements

WHO has many people to thank for the production of this advisory note of the WHO Study Group on Tobacco Product Regulation (TobReg). Ms Gemma Vestal coordinated the production, with the supervision and support of Dr Armando Peruga and Dr Douglas Bettcher.

Special appreciation goes to the contributors, who worked with us for a full year so that this advisory note could be launched during the Waterpipe Tri-Plenary at the 16th World Conference on Tobacco or Health, on 17–21 March 2015, in Abu Dhabi, United Arab Emirates. The contributors, Dr Elie Akl, Dr Thomas Eissenberg, Dr Wasim Maziak, Dr Purnima Mehrotra, Mr Jeremy Morton and Dr Alan Shihadeh, all worked tirelessly through many drafts and revisions.

Our infinite gratitude to all the members of TobReg for their full, wholehearted dedication, time and unfailing commitment to fulfilling their mandate to advise WHO on tobacco product regulation, a highly complex area of tobacco control. We thank them for the numerous hours they spent reviewing the manuscript and for their insightful advice and guidance. As independent experts, members of TobReg serve WHO without remuneration.

Administrative support throughout the months of production was provided by WHO colleagues Ms Miriamjoy Aryee-Quansah, Mr Gareth Burns, Ms Elaine Alexandre Caruana, Mr Luis Madge, Ms Elizabeth

Tecson, Ms Rosane Serrao and Ms Moira Sy.

Special thanks are due to Dr Ala Alwan, Regional Director of the WHO Eastern Mediterranean Region, and to his colleagues Dr Samer Jabbour, Director of the department for Noncommunicable Diseases and Mental Health, and Dr Fatimah El Awa, Regional Advisor for the Tobacco Free Initiative, for their vision and leadership in convening and hosting the workshop for preparation of this second edition at the Regional Office, on 30 and 31 March 2014 in Cairo, Egypt. At that meeting, the initial outline of the second edition and the terms of reference for each of the section contributors were decided. With the cooperation and flexibility of the contributors and TobReg members, the contents were subsequently reframed to address the requests made by the Conference of the Parties to the WHO FCTC at its sixth session, in October 2014 in Moscow, Russian Federation.

In addition, we would like to convey our appreciation to the WHO editor, copyeditor and proofreader and to the layout and typesetter company in Portugal for their eye for detail and their patience with the tight deadlines under which they worked. We also express our gratitude to Mr Jon Barnhart of Health Partners, LLC for creating the front cover image and Mr Christophe Oliver for the illustrations of the waterpipe from the Middle East and the "bong" waterpipe.

Last but not least, WHO expresses its profound gratitude to former interns at the Tobacco Free Initiative who contributed large amounts of their internship time to the fruition of this document: Ms Aurelie Abrial, Ms Hannah Patzke and Ms Angeli Vigo. It is our hope that they continue to work passionately in some aspect of tobacco control, whatever bright career they follow in the future.

Undoubtedly, many people to whom we are indebted are not mentioned here, because so many people were involved in production of this report. We apologize for any omission. We therefore thank both those who are named and those who are not named. Without your assistance and support, none of this would have been possible. Thank you very much.

3. Purpose

This advisory note from TobReg addresses growing concern about the increasing prevalence and potential health effects of tobacco smoking with waterpipes. The first edition of this advisory note was published almost a decade ago, in 2005 (*1*). During the intervening period, much research has been conducted on both the health hazards and the increasing prevalence of waterpipe smoking in many countries and populations. Despite the increase in knowledge, there is still a prevailing public misconception that waterpipe tobacco smoking is somehow protective or "safer" than cigarette smoking. In some countries, the prevalence of waterpipe tobacco smoking has increased in certain subgroups to exceed that of cigarette smoking.

Given these trends, more effort is needed to bring policy on waterpipe tobacco smoking into line with the WHO FCTC. The purposes of this advisory note are to provide guidance to WHO and its Member States, to inform regulatory agencies in implementing the provisions of the WHO FCTC concerning education and communications, to suggest policy and to inform consumers about the risks of waterpipe smoking. It also provides a more thorough understanding of the health effects of waterpipe tobacco smoking to researchers, research agencies and funding bodies. In addition, the advisory note addresses those engaged in tobacco smoking prevention and cessation programmes, to ensure that such programmes accommodate the unique aspects of waterpipe use.

4. Background and history

While there are numerous kinds of waterpipe around the world, the kind addressed in this note is popularly referred to as "*narghileh*", "*shisha*" or "*hookah*", the type globalized in the 1990s. It includes a head or tobacco bowl (in which tobacco is placed), a body, a water bowl, a hose and a mouthpiece (Figure 1). Holes in the bottom of the head allow smoke to pass into the body's central conduit, which is submerged in water (or alcohol or soft drinks), half-filling the water bowl. The leather or plastic hose exits from the top of the water bowl and terminates with a mouthpiece, from which the smoker inhales. Charcoal or a briquette[1] is placed on top of the tobacco-filled head, often separated from the tobacco by a perforated aluminium foil sheet. After the head or tobacco bowl is loaded and the charcoal lit, the smoker inhales through the hose, drawing air into and around the charcoal. The resulting heated air, which also contains charcoal combustion products, then passes through the tobacco, which, as it is heated, produces the mainstream smoke aerosol. The smoke passes through the waterpipe body, bubbles through the water in the bowl and is carried though the hose to the smoker. During a smoking session, smokers typically replenish and adjust the charcoal to maintain the desired taste and smoke concentration. A pile of lit charcoal may be

---

1 Briquettes are sometimes used instead of charcoal; hereafter, all references to charcoal include briquettes.

kept in a nearby firebox for this purpose, which may present an additional inhalation hazard. Smokers may opt for more convenient, easy-lighting briquettes, which can be lit directly with a portable lighter. Because of the communal nature of waterpipe smoking, with sharing of a mouthpiece, there is potential transmission of infectious diseases.

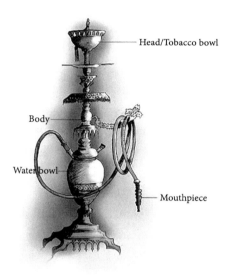

Head/Tobacco bowl

Body

Water bowl

Mouthpiece

Figure 1. A Middle-East waterpipe

There are regional and cultural differences in waterpipe design features, such as the size of the head or water bowl and the number of mouthpieces, but all waterpipes contain water through which smoke passes before reaching the smoker.

Waterpipes should be differentiated from the electronic devices known as "e-hookahs", "e-shisha" or "hookah pens". These devices are types of electronic nicotine delivery systems, which can be flavoured so that the taste is similar to that of the flavoured waterpipe tobacco called *maassel*. The electronic devices do not involve charcoal combustion; rather, a sweetened liquid is electrically heated to create an aerosol that is then inhaled. Research is currently being done on these devices.

Although cigarette smoking is the dominant form of tobacco use in most parts of the world, waterpipe use accounts for a significant and growing share of tobacco use globally. It is most prevalent in Asia, Africa and the Middle East, but it is a rapidly emerging problem on other continents. In the WHO Eastern Mediterranean Region, waterpipe use has surpassed cigarette use in some countries, with growing use by both men and women and, most seriously, among young people and children (2).

4.1 History

Waterpipes have been used to smoke tobacco and other substances, such as flowers, spices, fruits, coffee, marijuana or hashish, by the indigenous people of Africa and Asia for at least four centuries, and perhaps earlier (3). Their origin is somewhat nebulous, but it is known that trade routes through India and China helped disseminate the practice throughout parts of Asia, the Middle East and Africa (4). A form of waterpipe used in India in the sixteenth century was made from a coconut shell as the water reservoir, with a bamboo reed inserted through the top (4). This type of coconut-shell hookah was used by commoners, while smokers in affluent families used brass hookahs with ornate designs (5). According to one historical account (6), the waterpipe was invented in India by a physician during the reign of Emperor Akbar (who ruled from 1556 to 1605) as a purportedly less harmful method of tobacco use. The physician, Hakim Abul Fath, suggested that tobacco "smoke should be first passed through a small receptacle of water so that it would be rendered harmless." (5, 6) Thus, the widespread but unsubstantiated belief held by many waterpipe users today—that the practice is relatively safe— may be as old as the waterpipe itself (7).

4.2   Recent emergence

Waterpipes can be purchased from dedicated supply shops (including Internet vendors) that also sell charcoal, tobacco and accessories. Waterpipes are sometimes marketed as portable, with accessories such as carrying straps or cases. Some accessories are sold that are claimed to reduce the harmfulness of the smoke, such as mouthpieces containing activated charcoal or cotton, chemical additives to the water bowl and plastic mesh fittings to create smaller bubbles. None of these accessories has been tested empirically to verify whether they reduce smokers' exposure to toxicants or diminish their risks for tobacco-caused disease and death.

Misconceptions about the less harmful nature of waterpipes may be reinforced by marketing tools for the pipes and the tobacco. For example, the label of a popular waterpipe tobacco brand sold in several regions of the world states that it contains "0.5% nicotine and 0% tar". Others claim their product to be "natural" or "free of chemicals". Popular advertising shows waterpipes made from coconuts or pineapples. One advertisement states that not a single tree was cut down to make the product. Unlike cigarette packaging, which usually carries mandated health warnings, waterpipe tobacco products are commonly sold with no health warning.

Although waterpipe tobacco smoking had reportedly become associated with elderly men in the Middle East, in the 1990s, it quickly surged to become an epidemic among young people. This trend started in the Middle East and spread to universities and schools in many countries and continents. The increasing prevalence of waterpipe use outside regions in which it is traditionally known is reflected in the growth of the international waterpipe industry. The International Hookah Fair[2] is a trade fair showcasing the latest developments in waterpipes, hookah tobacco and similar products, with participants from over 60 countries. The evolution of these fairs reflects the demand for waterpipe products, with a continuous increase in both fair visitors and exhibitors since its establishment in 2013.

---

2   http://hookahfair.com/index.php/en/

5. Factors that contribute to the increase in prevalence and spread of use

It is hard to identify all the factors responsible for the global spread of an addictive behaviour such as waterpipe smoking. An addictive behaviour tends to spread gradually unless it is countered by effective policies and regulations. The focus of this advisory note is on the unique features of waterpipes and the combination of factors, within or outside the context of the waterpipe, that have contributed to its fast spread globally. These are: the introduction of flavoured tobacco, social acceptability due to the café and restaurant culture, developments in mass communication and social media and lack of waterpipe-specific policy and regulations.

5.1 Introduction of flavoured tobacco (*maassel*)

The definite date of the first production of sweetened flavoured waterpipe tobacco, commonly called *maassel*, is unknown, but it was already in use in the Middle East in the early 1990s (8). Circumstantial evidence suggests a temporal link between the production of *maassel* at the beginning of the 1990s and the surge in the number of waterpipe smokers in the Middle East (8). *Maassel* is typically manufactured by fermentation of tobacco with molasses, glycerine and fruit essence, producing a moist, pliable mixture. Before the introduction of *maassel*, most waterpipe smokers used some form of raw tobacco that they manipulated (e.g. crushed, mixed with water, squeezed and moulded) before use. This method usually produces strong, harsh smoke, unlike the smooth aromatic smoke produced from *maassel* (*9*). In retrospect, the introduction of *maassel* for waterpipes was the equivalent of the Bonsack machine, which enabled mass production and marketing of cigarettes. Industrialization and commercialization of *maassel* and its increased availability and variety made it appealing to young people, paving the way for mass marketing through the Internet, and simplified waterpipe preparation (*9*).

Data from all over the world show that *maassel* is the preferred tobacco for use in waterpipes by most smokers, especially young ones (*8–11*). For example, in a survey conducted in 2010 among 3447 students in eight universities in North Carolina (USA), 90% of students who had ever used a waterpipe smoked *maassel* (*11*). Many waterpipe smokers are drawn to this method because of the aromatic, smooth smoke and the variety of flavours of *maassel* (*12*).

5.2   Social acceptability due to the café and restaurant culture

The strong social dimension of waterpipe smoking has been well characterized (*9–14*). Many waterpipe smokers practise the habit in the company of friends and family, and it is a central component of social and family gatherings (*9, 10, 15, 16*). Sharing the same waterpipe is also a well-recognized, widespread practice, especially among young people (*9, 10, 17*). Lasting for an hour or more, at a relatively slow puffing rate, waterpipes are conducive to social interactions, especially in café settings. These features coincided with a boom in the café culture among young people in the Middle East and globally (*12*). One of the milestones in this regard was the introduction of "Ramadan tents" in the 1990s, which were a special form of café that provided a social venue during the Muslim holy month of Ramadan. Especially young people gathered in the evening after breaking their fast, and waterpipes became the centrepieces of such settings (*18*). They provided the nicotine for smokers (smoking is not allowed during fasting), an especially active social experience during Ramadan and lengthy sensory indulgence after the strict deprivation of fasting.

As waterpipes gained appeal among tourists and young people outside the Eastern Mediterranean region, expatriates from the region opened waterpipe cafés and restaurants around the world. The enterprise took on a life of its own, and waterpipe cafés began to open in most urban centres of the world, benefiting largely from the weak or absent regulatory framework for this tobacco use. In the USA for example, the number of hookah cafés has increased dramatically in the past decade, and they are often situated around university campuses (*17*). In a study of 3770 students in eight US universities, current waterpipe smoking was associated with the presence of a waterpipe café or restaurant within a 10-mile (16-km) radius of the university campus (*19*).

5.3   Developments in mass communication and social media

A local trend, such as waterpipe smoking in Middle Eastern societies, will either remain local or spread slowly in the absence of global communication and networking systems. The waterpipe epidemic has benefited from two technological developments. The first occurred in the 1990s, with the introduction of unregulated, inexpensive, widely accessible satellite television media throughout the Middle East. As a result, satellite television quickly became the entertainment of choice for the masses, and new satellite channels were launched constantly, with increasing air time to be filled. Social activities involving waterpipes, such as Ramadan tents, quickly found air time and were transmitted throughout the region (*18*).

The second technological innovation that probably contributed to the increasing popularity of waterpipe smoking among the young and educated was the Internet. This was particularly relevant to the spread of waterpipe use from the Middle East to regions with little or no knowledge of this form of tobacco use. In a recent study, trends in search engine queries about waterpipes were compared with trends in queries about electronic cigarettes between 2004 and 2013 in Australia, Canada, the United Kingdom and the USA. The study showed that Internet-based searches for waterpipes increased steadily in all four countries during the period and were more frequent for waterpipes than for e-cigarettes in Australia, Canada and the USA, the highest volume being documented in the USA (Figure 2) (*20*).

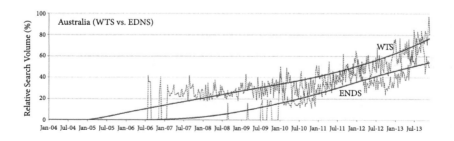

5. Factors that contribute to the increase in prevalence and spread of use

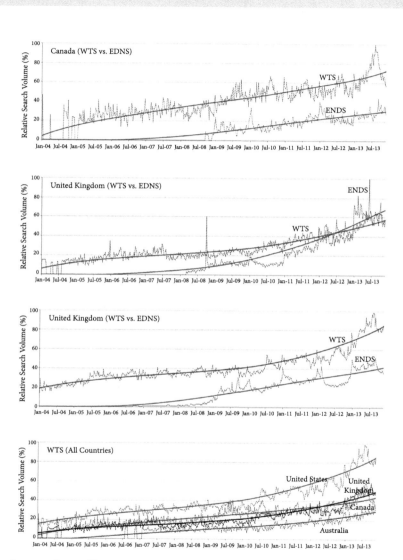

Source: reference *20*

WTS, waterpipe tobacco smoking; ENDS, electronic nicotine delivery system

Figure 2. Internet search patterns for waterpipe and e-cigarettes in Australia, Canada, the United Kingdom and the UsA

The online searches were primarily for waterpipe products for home use, followed by searches for waterpipe cafés and lounges. The largely unregulated Internet allows waterpipe promoters to circumvent most of the advertisement bans and reach their preferred customer pool of the young and educated. In an analysis of 144 websites of waterpipe venues in the USA, only 4% posted tobacco-related health warnings (21). A similar analysis of cigarette- and waterpipe-related YouTube videos showed that user-generated videos of waterpipe use were less likely to acknowledge the negative health consequences of smoking than cigarette videos. In fact, 92% of waterpipe-related videos and only 24% of cigarette-related videos portrayed smoking in a positive light (22). Much of the promotion on the Internet and in social media is portrayed as a front for interest groups but in fact disguises waterpipe sellers and marketers (e.g. www.hookahblogger. tumblr.com/ and www.hookah-shisha.com/hookahlove/) (21–23).

5.4   Lack of waterpipe-specific policy and regulations

Despite the remarkable success of public health policies in reducing cigarette smoking in many countries, waterpipe smoking has thrived in the wake of strict tobacco control policies and regulations that are mostly cigarette-oriented. For example, waterpipe venues and products in many developed countries are exempt from tobacco control policies, and lack of enforcement of relevant tobacco control policies is the main problem in developing countries. This has contributed to the proliferation of waterpipe venues all over the world (14, 24).

While cigarette pack size and packaging are fairly uniform worldwide, this is not the case for waterpipes. Waterpipes vary in shape and size, are less portable, comprise multiple parts, are often shared and involve diverse commercial stakeholders. Therefore, many policy-related elements must be waterpipe-specific (25). For example, a typical waterpipe smoker in a public venue does not see the tobacco package or the warning labels about the health risks associated with the use of tobacco, charcoal combustion or spread of infection (9, 26, 27). To address this limitation, Turkey has extended warning labelling to the bottles or bowls of waterpipes, requiring that warnings be placed on both sides of waterpipe bottles to cover 65% of the surface (2).

Whereas most price-based policies have been effective in curtailing the demand for cigarettes (28, 29), raising the price of *maassel* might not have the same effect, particularly with regard to waterpipe smoking in a café or restaurant, where tobacco constitutes only a small component of the profit margin (14). As anyone can prepare homemade *maassel* from relatively cheap ingredients,[3] waterpipe smokers may be less sensitive to price than cigarette smokers. Additionally, flavouring is considered a major factor in the appeal to young people, yet bans on the use of flavours in tobacco often do not cover waterpipe tobacco products.

This synopsis of the factors that contribute to widespread waterpipe smoking globally is based on an analysis of converging lines of evidence from different sources. While it is obviously limited, its aim is to increase understanding of the dynamics of the global waterpipe epidemic in order to control the spread (12).

---

3   http://www.thehookahlounge.org/how-to-make-your-own-shisha/, accessed 5 July 2014.

6. Regional and global patterns of waterpipe smoking

Waterpipe smoking has traditionally been associated with the Eastern Mediterranean region, Southeast Asia and northern Africa (*30–32*). Waterpipe use is, however, increasing globally (*1, 31, 33–37*), particularly among schoolchildren (*31, 38–46*) and university students (*33, 47, 48*). In many countries, waterpipe smoking is not monitored specifically; however, a systematic review of studies of the prevalence of waterpipe smoking in various populations and subpopulations showed alarmingly high numbers, especially among high-school and university students of Middle Eastern descent (*31*).

Several epidemiological studies have indicated the growing use of waterpipes in all WHO regions and among young people and adults of both genders. According to the Global Youth Tobacco Survey of tobacco use among 13–15-year-old children, use of tobacco products other than cigarettes increased in 34 of 100 sites surveyed, which was largely attributed to rising waterpipe use. The prevalence was 6–34% in the countries that reported data (*38*). Although nationally representative data on waterpipe use by adults are not widely available, the Global Adult Tobacco Survey showed that waterpipe smoking may be emerging in countries in which this tobacco product was not used previously (*34*). In this section, we present the epidemiology of waterpipe use in the six WHO regions.

6.1 African Region

Research on waterpipe use in Africa is limited. Three empirical studies in South Africa were conducted among students. In the first study, 60% of high-school students in a poor urban community in Johannesburg reported ever having used a waterpipe, while 20% reported daily use (*49*). The second study, among medical students in Pretoria, found that 19% of the participants had ever used a waterpipe (*50*). In the third study, conducted among university students in Western Cape, 40% of the participants reported current use of waterpipes, and, of these, 70% reported daily use (*51*). Almost half the users (48%) thought that the harmful effects of waterpipe smoking were greatly exaggerated. Waterpipe use fit the global pattern of the young embracing waterpipe smoking as a social experience.

In the Global Adult Tobacco Survey in Nigeria in 2012 (*52*), a very low prevalence was found of current use of tobacco products other than cigarette smoking (0.8% overall, 1.6% males, 0.1% females) in the entire population aged ⩾ 15 years. Although empirical evidence is lacking for other countries in this Region[4], anecdotal evidence for Algeria, Ethiopia, Kenya, Nigeria, Sudan, Uganda and the United Republic of Tanzania (*53*) indicates a proliferation of fashionable hookah bars in the larger urban centres in all these countries, which are frequented mainly by the young and business people.

---

4 The results of Global Adult Tobacco Surveys of waterpipe smoking in Cameroon, Senegal and Uganda were not available at the time of this publication.

6.2   Region of the Americas

Some research has been done and published on waterpipe tobacco smoking in Canada and the USA, but much less in the Latin American countries. A study in Canada showed that the prevalence of current and any use of waterpipes increased by 2.6% among young people between 2006 and 2010 (54). This trend was especially noticeable, as cigarette smoking among young people had significantly decreased in recent years. In the USA, the latest data on adults (aged $\geqslant$ 18 years) indicate prevalence rates of 0.5% for use every day and on some days and 3.9% for use every day, on some days and rarely, while use every day, on some days and rarely among 18–24-year-olds was 18.2% (55).

In a national study in the USA (56), of the 104 434 university students for whom complete information was available on cigarette, waterpipe and cigar use, 8733 (8.4%) were current waterpipe users. In this group, 4492 (51.4%) reported no current use of cigarettes, and 3609 (41.3%) reported no current use of other forms of tobacco. Of the 104 434 respondents, 31 794 (30.4%) had used a waterpipe at some time; of these, 9423 (29.7%) reported never using cigarettes, and 6198 (19.5%) reported never using tobacco of any kind. Thus, after cigarette smoking, waterpipe smoking was the most frequent form of tobacco use. Among adolescents, the rate of waterpipe smoking in the past month was 2.6% and that of any use was 7.3%. The authors concluded that "nearly one in five adolescents will try hookah before high-school graduation". A nationally representative study of high-school seniors showed an 18% rate of waterpipe use in the past year; those of a higher socioeconomic status were at particular risk for waterpipe smoking (*57*).

Significant waterpipe tobacco smoking does not appear to be common in Latin America, although the published literature is limited. The Global Adult Tobacco Survey showed very low rates in Brazil in 2008, Mexico in 2009, Uruguay in 2010 and Argentina in 2012, with an overall prevalence of < 0.2% in all four countries (*34*, *58*). The rates for young adults were similarly low.

6.3　Eastern Mediterranean Region

The Eastern Mediterranean Region (which includes Middle Eastern and North African countries) has the highest prevalence of waterpipe use in the world (*59*), especially among young people (*30–32, 60*). In a longitudinal study of smoking among young people in the Region in 2008–2010, the prevalence of waterpipe smoking increased by 40% within 2 years of follow-up (from 13.3% to 18.9%; $p < 0.01$) (*61*). In a representative study of 13–15-year-old schoolchildren in various countries in the Region, the prevalence of waterpipe smoking ranged from 9% to 15% (*62*). In these studies, the prevalence of waterpipe smoking was actually higher than that of cigarette smoking. A Global Youth Tobacco Survey showed that use of other tobacco products (mainly waterpipes) was more frequent than cigarette smoking among children aged 13–15 in all 17 countries of the Region (*38*).

Data on adults are available from the Global Adult Tobacco Surveys for Egypt (2009) (*63*) and Qatar (2013) (*64*). In the population aged ⩾ 15 years, the prevalence of waterpipe use was 6.2% for males and 0.3% for females in Egypt and 4.9% for males and 1.6% for females in Qatar. In

Egypt, the men who smoked waterpipes tended to be older (40–54 years), live in rural areas and be less educated, consistent with previous results, reflecting the old tradition of waterpipe smoking in Egypt (*34*).

6.4 European Region

According to the Global Adult Tobacco Survey, the overall current and daily prevalence of waterpipe smoking in the population aged ⩾ 15 years were lower than those of cigarette smoking. The prevalence among men was highest in the Russian Federation in 2009 (4.4%), followed by Turkey in 2008 (4.0%), Ukraine in 2010 (3.2%) and Romania in 2011 (0.3%) (*34, 65*). In these countries, users were young (18–24 years), lived in urban areas, were better educated and tended to be occasional rather than daily users (*34*).

According to a Eurobarometer report in 2012 on the prevalence of and attitudes to tobacco in the 28 countries of the European Union among people aged ⩾ 15 years (*35*), 16% reported that they had tried a waterpipe at least once, an increase over the prevalence found in the previous survey in 2009. Use of waterpipes was most widespread in Latvia (42%), Estonia (37%) and Lithuania (36%) and least prevalent in Ireland (5%), Portugal (5%), Malta (8%) and Spain (8%). The greatest percentage increases in waterpipe use were reported in Austria, the Czech Republic and Luxembourg, while the largest decrease was reported in Sweden. In general, young male respondents and students reported more waterpipe use.

Smaller-scale studies also showed increasing use of waterpipes in Europe. In the United Kingdom, the prevalence among university students was

8–11%, and that among secondary school students was 8% (*47, 66, 67*). In a study of 920 high-school students in France (mean age, 18 years), 40% reported experimenting with tobacco products other than cigarettes, including waterpipes (*68*). In a national study of 13 826 students in Estonia (aged 11–15 years), waterpipe use was reported by 25% of boys and 16% of girls (*69*). In a study of schoolchildren in Israel, 22% reported weekly use of waterpipes (*70*). Other studies in Israel also showed a high prevalence of waterpipe use among schoolchildren (< 18 years) (*71, 72*), up to 40% (*73*).

6.5   South-East Asia Region

Global Adult Tobacco Survey data collected between 2008 and 2011 on waterpipe use was available for Bangladesh and Thailand in 2009, India in 2010 and Indonesia in 2011 (*34, 74*). The prevalence among men was highest in Bangladesh (1.3%), followed by India (1.1%), Indonesia (0.3%) and Thailand (0.03%); the prevalence among women was highest in India (0.6%), followed by Bangladesh (0.2%), Thailand (0.01%) and Indonesia (0.0%). In India, the prevalence of waterpipe smoking was significantly higher in people aged > 50 years than in those aged < 30 years (2.0% vs 0.3%), in those living in rural rather than urban areas (1.1% vs 0.0%), in those with lower rather than higher educational attainment (1.4% vs 0.0%) and among current cigarette smokers than among non-cigarette smokers (5.6% vs 0.6%) (*75*).

No empirical evidence was available on the prevalence of waterpipe smoking in the other countries in the Region; however, anecdotal evidence from newspapers and online resources shows that hookah bars and restaurants are becoming increasingly common and are most often frequented by young people.

6.6　Western Pacific Region

There is a long history of smoking tobacco through "bong" waterpipes[5] (Figure 3) in Asia, which are different from traditional Arabic waterpipes (34) and are not usually included in research on waterpipe tobacco smoking. Bong waterpipes can be made of bamboo, metal or glass and are used in countries such as China, the Lao People's Democratic Republic, Myanmar and Viet Nam. They may be misconceived as less harmful than the Eastern Mediterranean hookah waterpipe (76).

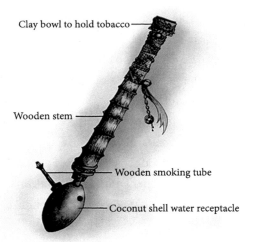

Clay bowl to hold tobacco

Wooden stem

Wooden smoking tube

Coconut shell water receptacle

Figure 3. A Chinese bong waterpipe

5　Bongs are slightly different from waterpipes used in the Middle East: the bong is not necessarily used with charcoal, perhaps resulting in less exposure to carbon monoxide.

In a comparison of 13 countries worldwide, the highest rate of waterpipe tobacco smoking among males (aged ⩾ 15 years) was found in Viet Nam in 2010 (13.0%), the rate being higher than that in Egypt in 2009 (6.2%) and in Turkey in 2008 (4.0%) (*34*). The highest prevalence of waterpipe smoking in Viet Nam was in older age groups (40–54 years), those living in rural areas and less educated people. The prevalence in Vietnamese women was very low (0.2%).

A Global Adult Tobacco Survey in China in 2010 showed a prevalence in the population aged ⩾ 15 years of only 0.65% for males and 0.08% for females. In a Global Adult Tobacco Survey in Malaysia in 2011, the prevalence in people aged ⩾ 15 years was 1.0% for males and 0.1% for females (*77*).

The traditional bong waterpipes thus appear to be used by older, rural, less educated men. There is anecdotal evidence, however, that many traditional Middle Eastern hookah cafés are opening in cities in the Region, and the prevalence of waterpipe tobacco smoking should be monitored as these cafés become more common. In the surveys cited above, no distinction was made between traditional Eastern Mediterranean waterpipes and bong waterpipes.

7. Health effects of the toxicant content of waterpipe smoke

As burning charcoal is usually used as the heat source in waterpipes, the smoke contains toxicants emitted from both the charcoal and the tobacco product, including flavourings. Thus, the composition of both the charcoal and the tobacco can influence the toxicant content of the smoke.

Laboratory studies during the past decade with the use of modern analytical methods and reliable machine smoke generation and sampling protocols have begun to elucidate the toxicant content of waterpipe smoke. Numerous carcinogens and toxicants have been identified, such as tobacco-specific nitrosamines, polycyclic aromatic hydrocarbons (PAH) (e.g. benzo[a]pyrene, anthracene), volatile aldehydes (e.g. formaldehyde, acetaldehyde, acrolein), benzene, nitric oxide and heavy metals (arsenic, chromium, lead). The charcoal contributes to high levels of carbon monoxide (CO) and the generation of carcinogenic PAH (2). Some of these chemicals are classified by the International Agency for Research on Cancer (IARC) as human carcinogens (78). In 2014, it was reported that people exposed to waterpipe smoke are at risk for leukaemia due to benzene uptake (79).

Additional factors that influence the toxicant content of the waterpipe smoke aerosol are puff topography (i.e. the number of puffs drawn, the puff volume, duration of puffs and the interval between consecutive puffs) and waterpipe design and construction. Waterpipes are not standardized, although some attempt has been made to standardize them, and they therefore vary in numerous ways, including the volume of the head space above the water and the porosity of the hose through which the user draws smoke. Differences in hose porosity can greatly influence the toxicant content, by varying dilution and combustion conditions (80).

Published reports on the toxicant content of waterpipe smoke thus refer to a particular combination of charcoal and tobacco and specific waterpipe features and puffing parameters. In the same way as for cigarette smoke, reports on the toxicant content of waterpipe smoke vary widely. Nevertheless, all the studies to date indicate that, during a typical waterpipe use session, the user will draw large doses of toxicants (ranging from less than one to tens of cigarette equivalents) (Figure 4). These toxicants have been linked to addiction, heart and lung diseases, and cancer in cigarette smokers and can result in similar outcomes in waterpipe users if these toxicants are absorbed in the body in appreciable amounts.

The nicotine in waterpipe products is responsible for their dependence potential (addictiveness). For a single smoking session of 10 g of *maassel* tobacco with 1.5 quick-lighting charcoal discs applied to the waterpipe head, 2.94 mg nicotine, 802 mg "tar" and 145 mg CO were measured in the mainstream smoke (2).

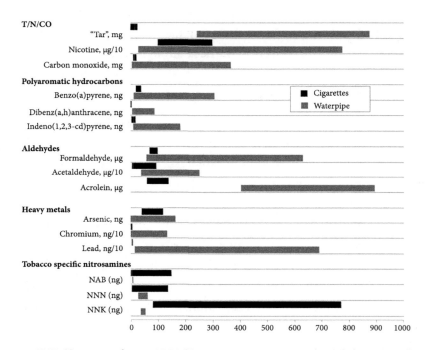

NAB, *N*-nitrosoanabasine; NNN, *N*-nitrosonornicotine; NNK, (4-methylnitrosamino)-1-(3-pyridyl)-1-butanone Data on cigarettes from Apsley et al. (*81*) and Jenkins et al. (*82*) and data on waterpipes from Monzer et al. (*83*), Schubert et al. (*84*) and Shihadeh (*85*)

Figure 4. Reported ranges of toxicants produced during a single 1-h session of waterpipe use (in red) and from a single cigarette (in black)

7.1 Toxicant uptake by waterpipe users

While analyses of waterpipe smoke show clearly that it contains large doses of toxicants, they do not reveal whether the toxicants are absorbed by the smoker in appreciable amounts. Thus, another line of inquiry for assessing the potential hazard of waterpipe use is to study biomarkers of exposure to toxicants in the blood and urine of users. Such studies have been conducted to investigate acute, "multi-day" and long-term exposure to CO, nicotine, PAH or tobacco-specific nitrosamines (86–91). Waterpipe smoking results in significant exposure to all these compounds, and waterpipe smokers have much greater exposure to CO, significantly greater exposure to PAH, similar exposure to nicotine and significantly lower exposure to tobacco-specific nitrosamines than cigarette smokers (87, 91). These findings are consistent across studies and mirror the pattern of differences found in analyses of the toxicant content of waterpipe and cigarette smoke. Even when the results are normalized for nicotine, waterpipe smoke contains much more CO, more PAH and less tobacco-specific nitrosamines than cigarette smoke. Comparison of exposure biomarkers in the blood and urine of waterpipe and cigarette smokers reflects this pattern.

7.2   Acute physiological and health effects of waterpipe use

Waterpipe use has deleterious effects on the respiratory system, cardiovascular system, oral cavity and teeth, and long-term waterpipe smokers have higher incidences of chronic obstructive pulmonary disease and periodontal disease (2, 92).

The emission of high levels of CO leads to syncope among some users due to CO intoxication secondary to the formation of carboxyhaemoglobin in blood, which compromises the transport of sufficient oxygen to body parts, including the brain (2). Acute CO poisoning of waterpipe users has also been reported (93, 94), and acute effects have been reported in several controlled clinical studies. Some of the effects, such as elevated heart rate and blood pressure, are consistent with well-known effects of nicotine (95–97). Other deleterious acute cardiovascular effects, such as impaired baroreflex control (98) and cardiac autonomic dysfunction (87, 88), have also been documented and found to be independent of nicotine content. Waterpipe smoking also appears to impair lung function and exercise capacity (99) and to elicit changes in inflammation biomarkers (96). These effects are consistent with the notion that waterpipe smoke delivers physiologically active doses of not only nicotine but also other toxicants and suggest that chronic waterpipe use may lead to disease in the long term.

7.3   Second-hand waterpipe smoke

Second-hand smoke emitted directly from waterpipes into the surrounding atmosphere also contains toxicants, as shown in controlled laboratory test chambers (100, 101) and by measurement of airborne particulate matter in settings where waterpipes are used (102–104). Collectively, these studies show that waterpipe smoking results in significant emissions of CO, aldehydes, PAH, ultrafine particles and respirable particulate matter. Establishments in which waterpipes are smoked exclusively tend to have higher concentrations of respirable particulate matter than those in which cigarettes are smoked exclusively (102, 103). On a smoker–hour basis, waterpipe smoking results in higher emissions of CO, PAH and volatile aldehydes than cigarette smoking (105). In addition, the direct emissions of toxicants from waterpipes smoked with a tobacco-free preparation were equal to or greater than those from waterpipes smoked with tobacco-based preparations. Thus, except for nicotine, smoke from tobacco-free waterpipe products has the same toxicant content and biological activity as that from tobacco-based products (*103*). These studies indicate that waterpipe smoking should be included in all regulations designed to minimize exposure to second-hand smoke.

7.4   Long-term health effects

A systematic review of the health effects of waterpipe tobacco smoking showed significant associations between waterpipe tobacco smoking and lung cancer, periodontal disease and low birth weight (*106*). The evidence available at that time (2010) was not sufficient to rule out or confirm associations with other outcomes, including other types of cancer. Since that review, more than 20 new, relevant studies have been published, which have contributed to the evidence base and to better understanding of the effects of waterpipe tobacco smoking on health, as detailed below.

Evidence available as of June 2014 suggested that waterpipe tobacco smoking is probably associated with the following types of cancer: oral cancer, with an odds ratio of about 4, based on two cross-sectional studies conducted in India and Yemen (*107, 108*); oesophageal cancer, with an odds ratio of 2.65, based on three case–control studies in the Islamic Republic of Iran and Kashmir (India) (*109–111*) and lung cancer, with an odds ratio of 2.12, based on six studies conducted in China,[6] India and Tunisia (*112–117*).

Waterpipe tobacco smoking may also be associated with gastric carcinoma, as suggested by a case–control study and a prospective cohort study, both

---

6   Although Chinese waterpipes are different from that shown in Figure 1. See Figure 3.

conducted in the Islamic Republic of Iran (*118*, *119*), and with urinary bladder cancer, as suggested by two case–control studies conducted in Egypt (*120*, *121*). During the past 5 years, significant evidence has become available for an association between waterpipe tobacco smoking and respiratory disease, mainly chronic bronchitis. A meta-analysis of data from five studies conducted in the Middle East and North Africa gave a pooled odds ratio of about 2 (*122–126*). In addition, cigarette smoking and waterpipe smoking have a synergistic effect on chronic obstructive pulmonary disease (*127*). A study of Chinese waterpipe smoking showed a significant increase in the risk for chronic obstructive pulmonary disease among waterpipe smokers and also among women exposed to second-hand waterpipe smoke (odds ratio, > 10) (*76*). It is important to recall that this disease is often associated with lung cancer (*128*).

In terms of cardiovascular disease, in a study of 1210 patients in four hospitals in Lebanon, those who had smoked waterpipes for > 40 years had a three times higher odds ratio for severe stenosis (> 70%) than non-smokers (odds ratio, 2.95; 95% confidence interval, 1.04–8.33) after adjustment for demographic characteristics and risk factors for coronary artery disease: cigarette smoking, alcohol consumption, insufficient physical activity, diabetes, hypertension, hyperlipidaemia and a family history of coronary artery disease (*129*). Another large prospective study, in Bangladesh, suggested that waterpipe tobacco smoking was associated with a 20% increase in mortality from ischaemic heart disease and stroke in men (*130*). A cross-sectional study in the Islamic Republic of Iran provided less conclusive evidence on the association between waterpipe tobacco smoking and self-reported heart disease but showed a dose–effect relation (i.e. a higher risk with higher exposure), making the association more likely (*131*). A few studies have addressed surrogate outcomes, such as the severity of findings on cardiac angiography, with results consistent with those described above (*129, 132*).

Three cross-sectional studies conducted in Egypt did not show an association between waterpipe use and hepatitis C infection (*133–135*). While there have been case reports of an association with tuberculosis (*27, 136, 137*), no formal study of the association has been published so far.

The association between waterpipe tobacco smoking and quality of life was assessed in two studies. A national cross-sectional study in Lebanon did not provide conclusive evidence of an association with "respiratory quality of life"[7] (*138*), while a similar study in the Islamic Republic of Iran found that people who smoked waterpipes reported poorer health-related quality of life (*139*).

Waterpipe tobacco smoking has been associated with a variety of other outcomes. Two retrospective cohort studies conducted in Lebanon and one case–control study in the Islamic Republic of Iran found an association between waterpipe tobacco smoking and low birth weight, with an odds ratio of about 2 (*140–142*). One cohort study in Egypt and four cross-sectional studies in Saudi Arabia consistently showed statistically significant associations with periodontal disease (*143–147*).

There have been isolated reports of associations between waterpipe use

---

7   Significant predictors of respiratory quality of life, in decreasing order of importance, are: cumulative number of cigarettes smoked, older age, having at least one smoker in the family, shorter education, female gender, living in a house heated with fuel oil, cumulative dose of smoke from waterpipe tobacco, living in a house heated with hot air and working with at least one smoker.

and other health effects. One cross-sectional study in Lebanon found an association between waterpipe smoking and perennial rhinitis (*148*); a study in Egypt suggested an association with male infertility (*49*); a large cross-sectional study in the Islamic Republic of Iran suggested an association with gastro-oesophageal reflux disease (*149*); and a national survey of university students in the USA found a moderate, statistically significant association between waterpipe smoking and poorer mental health (*150*).

7.5   Addiction to waterpipes

One of the main features of waterpipe smoking is the distinctive use pattern (*7*). Among young people in particular, waterpipe smoking is frequently practised as a group pastime, in the company of friends and family. A waterpipe smoking session takes an average of 1 h, and its limited accessibility or mobility contributes to the predominant pattern being intermittent use (*7*). Furthermore, there is a common misperception that the water has a filtering effect. These features indicate why many waterpipe smokers claim that it is not as addictive as cigarettes (*151*). Whether waterpipe smoking is as addictive as cigarettes at equal levels of use is not known, but evidence of the addictive nature of waterpipe smoking is accumulating and becoming unequivocal.

In 1997, Macaron and colleagues first showed the exposure of waterpipe smokers to nicotine, by measuring cotinine in their urine (*152*); this finding has been replicated repeatedly since. For example, in a recent laboratory study at the Syrian Centre for Tobacco Studies, waterpipe smokers who had been abstinent for 24 h were invited to the clinical laboratory for one session of waterpipe smoking while their venous blood was sampled for later analysis of nicotine. Waterpipe smoking led to about a fivefold increase in plasma nicotine levels (from 3.07 ± 3.05 ng/mL before smoking to 15.7 ± 8.7 ng/mL after smoking; $p < 0.001$) (153). In another study, the exposure of waterpipe and cigarette smokers to nicotine was compared in a two-condition cross-over design (i.e. if the first session was with a waterpipe, the second was with a cigarette and vice versa). While peak plasma nicotine levels did not differ in the two conditions, the dynamics of exposure and cumulative dose of nicotine were different, with a slower rise and more protracted, larger cumulative exposure for the waterpipe smokers than for the cigarette smokers (Figure 5) (154).

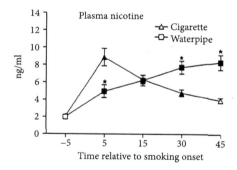

While both waterpipe and cigarette smoking were allowed ad libitum, the waterpipe was available for 45 min, and the cigarette was smoked in approximately 5 min. Filled symbols indicate a significant difference from baseline (time 0), and asterisks (*) indicate a significant difference between conditions at that time ($p < 0.001$).

Figure 5. Mean (± 1 standard error of the mean) plasma nicotine concentration in 31 participants who smoked tobacco using a waterpipe (triangles) or a cigarette (squares) in a laboratory session

Other than the neuropharmacological aspect of addiction mediated by nicotine, behavioural studies indicate dependence among waterpipe smokers, such as failed quit attempts, self-perception of being "hooked" on the waterpipe, use escalation over time, behavioural adaptation to ensure access and abstinenceinduced withdrawal that is suppressed by subsequent use (*33*). For example, in a random sample of 268 waterpipe users in Aleppo, Syria, 28% wanted to quit and 59% had made an unsuccessful attempt to quit in the past year. Belief in the ability to quit was inversely related to perceived dependence (*155*). This experience was confirmed in a standardized laboratory environment, in which waterpipe smokers who had been abstinent for 24 h were invited to the clinical laboratory of the Syrian Centre for Tobacco Studies to smoke a waterpipe *ad libitum*, and their subjective withdrawal and craving were measured before and after smoking. The results showed that the urge to smoke, restlessness, craving and other symptoms of abstinence were intense before smoking and were significantly reduced after smoking, while feeling dizzy or lightheaded and other direct effects of nicotine showed the opposite trend (*156*).

Personal interviews with waterpipe tobacco smokers reveal much about the addictiveness of this form of smoking. For example, a qualitative study brought out several interesting statements from waterpipe smokers: "I started smoking [waterpipe] when I was young and I know its side effects and I know what it does to my lungs. I go up the stairs, I start panting. But I cannot [stop it] because I am addicted to it, I would not mind stopping it but I cannot"; "I like to dominate everything, but the narghile [waterpipe] has completely dominated me. That bothers me. My happiness is related to the narghile. It is essential for having a good time…"; "I usually smoke narghile once daily, but sometimes I smoke more. Because even when I have already smoked it, seeing or smelling narghile makes me feel that I need to smoke again, and I usually do smoke" (*157*). These findings are consistent with the notion that waterpipe smoking is associated with features of tobacco and nicotine dependence similar to those associated with cigarette smoking.

While many of the indicators of waterpipe dependence are seen with cigarette smoking, there are strong reasons to believe that the unique features of waterpipes influence the development and manifestations of tobacco dependence in users. Waterpipe sharing, its social dimension and its limited accessibility are not usually covered in conventional models of tobacco dependence (*7*). Moreover, because a waterpipe is usually used repeatedly, even the act of purchasing one might be a more significant milestone than buying a pack of cigarettes. Nevertheless, studies of waterpipe dependence have relied so far on models and measures derived from the literature on cigarettes, which can lead to insufficient and erroneous judgements about the addictive potential of waterpipe smoking. For example, doubt was cast on the addictive nature of waterpipe smoking in a recent publication on the basis of the lack of evidence of a desire to smoke a waterpipe within the first 30 min of waking, which is a strong predictive measure of tobacco dependence in cigarette smokers (*158*). Such a critique is pointless in view of the known pattern of waterpipe smoking, with long smoking sessions in a relaxed atmosphere and social context. Almost a decade ago, waterpipe experts warned about the use of cigarette-specific scales or items (such as smoking within the first 30 min of waking) for assessing waterpipe dependence because of its incompatibility with known patterns of waterpipe use (*159*).

Evidence of the addictive potential of waterpipe smoking has spurred efforts to develop specific measures of tobacco dependence. One of the pioneer efforts was the Lebanon Waterpipe Dependence Scale (*160*). While this scale was not based on data for waterpipe smokers but was derived from the criteria of the Fagerström test for nicotine dependence and the *Diagnostic statistical manual of mental disorders* (4th revised edition), it has been used in several studies to measure dependence in waterpipe smokers (*161–163*). With this caveat, tobacco dependence in waterpipe smokers has unique features that continue to be unrecognized in models and instruments derived from the literature on cigarettes. Some of these features probably influence all stages of the development of dependence in waterpipe smokers. Thus, while the specific waterpipe cues of smell and sound may attract new users and reinforce use by established smokers, behavioural adaptation to ensure access may signify more advanced dependence. Daily smokers who perceive themselves to be addicted to waterpipes can engage in more intensive behavioural adaptations to ensure access, such as carrying their own waterpipe and selecting cafés on the basis of waterpipe availability (*37*).

The role of waterpipe-specific cues in attracting new smokers and supporting use has been demonstrated in several studies (*162*). For example, a recent qualitative study conducted in Lebanon supports the contribution of features like smell, sound and taste to young people's connection to the waterpipe (*18*). Specifically, the taste and smell of waterpipe tobacco (*maassel*) were listed as the main reasons for trying a waterpipe and eventually becoming addicted by some people: "my parents used to sit and smoke the waterpipe .... Then, from its nice smell we got hooked". The smell of the waterpipe, even in public places, motivated initiation of waterpipe smoking for some: "When you arrive at a café, you smell the waterpipe from the outside, you say that's it, you want to smoke it". Furthermore, studies on the attitudes and behaviour of waterpipe smokers in the Eastern Mediterranean Region and elsewhere repeatedly identified the influence of features such as the aromatic smell, the smooth taste of the smoke and the bubbling sound of water in shaping the waterpipe experience (*10, 12, 33, 152, 162, 164*). These unique features of waterpipe use and its associative cues to smokers require a novel approach to prevention and cessation of waterpipe use based on evidence from research on the development and character of the dependence of waterpipe smokers and the factors that influence it.

7.6　Waterpipes as a bridge to cigarette smoking

Another worrisome aspect of the spread of waterpipe smoking is its potential to thwart cessation attempts by adult cigarette smokers and to serve as a gateway to cigarette smoking among young people. Several lines of evidence support this potential. First, studies of smoking cessation in the Eastern Mediterranean Region have shown that some people who have quit cigarettes switch to waterpipes, perhaps to sate their craving and avoid withdrawal (*165*). The potential of waterpipes to replace cigarettes for abstinent cigarette smokers was investigated further in a clinical laboratory study in which dual waterpipe and cigarette smokers who had been abstinent for 12 h attended two randomly ordered sessions (waterpipe or cigarette) separated by 48 h. For both methods of tobacco use, the scores for withdrawal and craving were high at the beginning of the session (before smoking) and were significantly and comparably reduced during smoking either a cigarette or a waterpipe (Figure 6) (*166*).

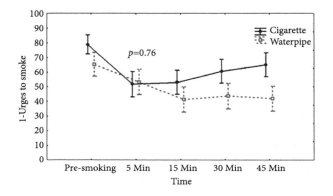

$p = 0.8$ for a comparison at 5 min in repeat-model analysis of variance

Figure 6. Mean scores for the item "Urge to smoke" in abstinent dual cigarette–waterpipe smokers

Qualitative studies of adult smokers extend this observation, showing that waterpipe use among cigarette quitters not only helps deal with abstinence symptoms but can increase the probability of failure of quit attempts. For example, in the qualitative study of adult waterpipe and cigarette smokers, one smoker stated "I quit smoking [cigarettes] for more than 6 months. Then, I was invited to smoke narghile [waterpipe]. After the second puff I asked for a cigarette and I started again" (*157*).

While such observations are indicative of the potential of waterpipes to replace and act as a bridge to cigarette smoking, the gateway hypothesis that waterpipe smoking leads to cigarette smoking is still being investigated. Generally, because of their size and the time-consuming preparation process, waterpipes are less accessible to smokers than cigarettes. These features are limiting for an addictive behaviour that requires frequent dosing, which led to the suggestion that young people who start their tobacco use with a waterpipe may turn to the more readily accessible cigarettes to deal with their dependence needs more rapidly (33). In other words, the balance between dependence and access may determine which waterpipe users are likely to initiate cigarette smoking. This hypothesis was tested in a longitudinal study of adolescents (aged 13 at baseline) who were not waterpipe or cigarette smokers at baseline and who were compared with people who had never smoked in terms of risk for future cigarette smoking. The 12-month risk of waterpipe smokers for initiating cigarette smoking was twice that of people who had never smoked, and the risk was dose-dependent (Figure 7) (167).

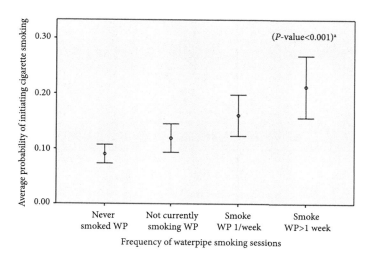

WP, waterpipe

Figure 7. 12-month average predicted probabilities of initiating cigarette smoking as a function of previous year's frequency of waterpipe smoking in a school-based sample of 1454 adolescents in irbid, Jordan, 2008–2011

These results strongly support the possibility that waterpipe smoking serves as a gateway to cigarette smoking and suggest the plausibility of the concept that more frequent (dependent) smokers are more likely to turn to cigarettes (*168*).

In summary, in order to deal effectively with waterpipe dependence, a waterpipespecific model and measures are needed to capture the full spectrum of experiences of waterpipe users at different stages of their smoking trajectory. Clear understanding is also needed of the role of environmental factors (e.g. policy, family, culture) and cigarette smoking in propagating waterpipe use. Such knowledge could guide waterpipe-specific prevention and intervention strategies to curb its global spread.

8. Research needs

The widespread use of waterpipe tobacco smoking across the globe and the many toxicants to which users are demonstrably (*86, 90*) or probably (*169*) exposed provide ample justification for vigorous research on the health risks associated with this form of tobacco use and on methods for preventing and treating it. There has been remarkable progress in some research areas, and this document shows that we have come closer to understanding national and global trends in waterpipe tobacco smoking; methods for evaluating toxicant yields; smokers' exposure to and absorption of toxicants; individual patterns of smoking; the relations among yield, exposure and absorption; and the pharmacology and toxicology of waterpipe smoke. During the past 10 years, research on waterpipe use has increased dramatically, especially in Germany, Jordan, Lebanon, the United Kingdom and the USA, but more is needed (*170, 171*). Progress is, however, slow, because individual research groups tend to work in relative isolation.

The global response to repeated calls for more research on all aspects of waterpipe tobacco smoking (*164, 172*) has been positive, but more must be done. A coordinated approach is required to address the critical research needs listed below.

- the types and patterns of waterpipe smoking in all regions and cultures (*1*);
- the extent to which the chemical and physical properties of the smoke

depend on the waterpipe set-up and smoking conditions (*1*);

- the epidemiology of waterpipe-associated acute health effects and disease risk, including addiction, transmission of non-tobacco-related communicable diseases (*1*), respiratory cancer and cardiovascular and other tobacco-related diseases, with an emphasis on understanding how patterns of use (for example, frequency, ingredients or material placed in the head and/or the bowl of the waterpipe, group versus individual sessions and whether the mouthpiece is shared) influence disease risk, taking into account specific groups, such as pregnant women and women of reproductive age;

- development of standardized biomarkers of exposure and effect, such as DNA adducts, in order to obtain complementary evidence of the biological effects of waterpipe smoke on cells and in experimental animals to determine whether waterpipe smoke induces inflammatory and oxidative stress responses;

- the influence of cultural and social practices on initiation and maintenance (*1*);

- the relation between smoking waterpipes and other forms of tobacco, including substitution and smoking multiple products (*1*), and the extent to which initiation of waterpipe tobacco smoking is a factor in subsequent use of other forms of tobacco;

- the relation between waterpipe tobacco smoking and use of other drugs, including marijuana (*1*);

- development of culturally relevant prevention and cessation strategies (*1*);

- development of measures of nicotine and tobacco dependence that are validated for waterpipe tobacco smoking, also taking into account differences in culture and language;

- the extent to which flavoured tobacco, waterpipe cafés and other marketing tools, economic factors and the absence of waterpipe-specific tobacco regulation influence the global spread of waterpipe tobacco smoking;

- the effect on non-smokers of exposure to waterpipe tobacco smoke and smoking, including health effects, and "renormalization" of tobacco smoking;

- experimental research on the effects of clinical and public health interventions on preventing and cessation of waterpipe tobacco smoking;

- whether use of waterpipes without tobacco or with very low-nicotine tobacco leads to dependence;

- epigenomic effects of waterpipe tobacco smoking, such as in the human respiratory epithelia;

- the role of flavours in increased initiation, dual use and continuation of use of other tobacco products, as well as long-term effects of flavours; and,

- for the WHO Tobacco Laboratory Network (TobLabNet),[8] assessment within 2 years of whether the standard operating procedures for measuring nicotine (*173*), tobacco-specific nitrosamines (*174*) and benzo[*a*]pyrene (*175*) in cigarette contents and emissions are applicable or adaptable as appropriate to waterpipe smoke, pursuant to the request to WHO at the sixth session of the Conference of the Parties to the WHO FCTC (*176*).

---

8   http://www.who.int/tobacco/industry/product_regulation/toblabnet/en/

9. Scientific basis and conclusions

While the evidence base for the health effects of waterpipe tobacco smoking remains sparse, it is nonetheless sufficient to justify strong control measures to limit the spread of this practice. As outlined above, every study to date has found that waterpipe tobacco smoke contains ample quantities of the toxicants known to cause diseases in cigarette smokers, including cancer, and that at least some of those toxicants are effectively absorbed by waterpipe users and are therefore present in their breath, blood and urine (177). A complementary line of evidence is derived from studies of the biological effects of waterpipe smoke on cells and experimental animals, which have shown that it induces inflammatory and oxidative stress responses (178) and plausible mechanisms for the development of vascular disease and chronic obstructive pulmonary disease in regular waterpipe users. The findings of epidemiological studies are congruent with those of toxicological research. The accumulating body of evidence shows that waterpipe tobacco smoking is probably associated with oral, oesophageal and lung cancers and possibly with gastric and bladder cancers. There is also evidence of associations with respiratory disease, cardiovascular disease, periodontal disease, low birth weight, perennial rhinitis, male infertility, gastro-oesophageal reflux disease and impairment of mental health (91). Uncertainty remains about an association with tuberculosis.

In summary, all the evidence, from studies of molecules to studies of human populations, converges towards the conclusion that waterpipe tobacco smoking causes diseases that are commonly associated with cigarette smoking, including addiction. While there are fewer studies of waterpipe tobacco smoke constituents and their biological activity and health effects than of cigarette smoke, the consistency of the evidence within and across scientific approaches suggests strongly that this basic conclusion will not change as more evidence becomes available. In light of the widespread, growing use of waterpipes worldwide, firm action is necessary and justified to protect public health.

10. Policy

At the sixth Conference of the Parties to the WHO FCTC, held in Moscow, Russian Federation, on 13–18 October 2014, WHO was invited to prepare a report on policy options and best practices in controlling use of waterpipe tobacco products in light of the WHO FCTC, to be submitted to the seventh session of the Conference of the Parties in November 2016 (*179*). TobReg hereby makes the following policy recommendations.

WHO FCTC article	specific policy recommendations for waterpipes
Article 5	**General obligations.** Even in countries with well-established tobacco control programmes, waterpipe tobacco smoking may be underrepresented or exempted because of its novelty in some countries and its long-standing traditional presence in others. Legislation and regulations on tobacco should specify all tobacco, not just in cigarettes, and should ensure that waterpipe-specific stipulations[9] are included in legislation in countries with a high or increasing prevalence.
Article 5.3	**Protection from vested commercial interests.** International exhibitions have been held recently to promote waterpipe tobacco products and accessories (*1*). Transparency should be required from waterpipe tobacco and accessory companies that are advocating for and against legislation and regulation, both directly and through third parties. No matter what role the tobacco industry plays in the production, distribution and sale of waterpipes and waterpipe products, this industry, its allies and front groups can never be considered a legitimate public health partner or stakeholder while it continues to profit from tobacco and its products or to represent its interests.

---

9   Waterpipes with or without tobacco in the "head"

Article 6	**Price and tax measures to reduce the demand for tobacco.** Because tax measures have been shown to reduce tobacco consumption, especially by young people, Parties should implement both tax and price measures on waterpipe tobacco and waterpipe products.
Article 8	**Protection from exposure to tobacco smoke.** Because all second-hand tobacco smoke has the potential to cause death, disability and disease, waterpipes should be included with cigarettes in clean indoor air policies. Waterpipe cafés or lounges should not be exempt from clean indoor air legislation.
Articles 9 and 10	**Regulation of the contents of tobacco products and tobacco product disclosures.** Policy should be implemented to ensure that waterpipe tobacco is included in legislation requiring the testing and regulation of tobacco contents and emissions, as well as the reporting thereof.
Article 11 a	**Health claims.** Waterpipe tobacco packaging and all waterpipe parts and accessories must not promote any misleading understanding about tobacco or give an erroneous view of the dangers inherent in its use.
b	**Health warnings.** Waterpipe tobacco, product packaging and waterpipes themselves should be labelled with health warnings in accordance with Article 11 of the WHO FCTC.
Article 12	**Education, awareness and training.** Given the prevalence of misinformation surrounding the health dangers of waterpipe tobacco smoking, specific education and training must be included in wider tobacco education and public awareness programmes implemented by Parties.
Article 13	**Advertising, promotion and sponsorship.** A comprehensive ban on advertising, promotion and sponsorship of waterpipes should be included under Article 13 of the WHO FCTC. Parties not in a position to undertake a comprehensive ban should strongly restrict such advertising, promotion and sponsorship.
Article 14	**Demand reduction measures concerning tobacco dependence and cessation.** In accordance with the measures listed in Article 14 of the WHO FCTC and the guideline, Parties should include waterpipe tobacco smoking in cessation and treatment programmes for tobacco dependence.
Article 15	**Illicit trade in tobacco products.** Legislation and measures prohibiting illicit trade in tobacco should follow the guidelines set forth in Article 15 of the WHO FCTC and should ensure that waterpipe tobacco is included with cigarettes and all other forms of tobacco.

Article 16	**Sales to and by minors.** Sales of all tobacco, including waterpipe tobacco, should be prohibited to minors under Article 16 of the WHO FCTC. Waterpipe venues should not be an exception to this legislation.
Additionally	**Product design and information.** Waterpipes and waterpipe products should be regulated to: –minimize the content and emissions of toxicants; –ensure that any nicotine used is of pharmacological quality; –minimize acute nicotine toxicity; –minimize CO toxicity from heated charcoal; –impede product alteration to include other drugs; –ban waterpipe tobacco with alcohol and sweet-like flavours that may appeal to children and young people; –require manufacturers and importers to disclose to government authorities information about the contents and emissions of waterpipe tobacco smoking; and –require registration of manufacturers and importers with govern-ment authorities.
	Surveillance and monitoring. It is recommended that governments use or strengthen existing tobacco surveillance and monitoring systems to assess the current prevalence and the evolution of waterpipe use in various demographic groups, including by gender and age.
	Assessment of fire risk. The use of charcoal poses a regulatory challenge regarding its contribution to fires, which should also be assessed, and Parties should consider establishing monitoring systems for that purpose (1).

11. Suggested actions for regulators

TobReg also recommends specific actions for regulators (*179*):

WHO FCTC Article	suggested actions for regulators
Article 6 a	In order to conform to Article 6 of the WHO FCTC, Parties should both implement tax measures on tobacco products and restrict or prohibit importation and sale of duty-free tobacco and waterpipe products.
b	The goal of tobacco taxation is to decrease demand by discouraging purchasers by cost. Therefore, the tax should actually be prohibitive. If waterpipe tobacco is taxed only in bulk (e.g. by kg), it is still relatively inexpensive for individual users. Parties should consider taxing waterpipe tobacco per individual serving or at higher bulk prices.
c	Waterpipes themselves, as well as parts and accessories, should also be taxed.
d	Waterpipes, waterpipe tobacco, parts and accessories should be prohibited or restricted from being sold tax- or duty-free.
Article 8	Waterpipe cafés or lounges must not be exempted from clean indoor air laws, as they are in some countries where waterpipes are traditionally smoked. Indoor waterpipe smoking in public areas should be prohibited and smoking allowed only outside. Waterpipe venues should not be allowed within large shopping areas, such as indoor malls.
Articles 9 and 10	Waterpipe tobacco and waterpipe smoke should be tested by the same stringent standards that are applied to cigarette tobacco. Legislation should ensure that waterpipe tobacco is not exempt from testing and regulation of contents and emissions. The results of the testing of contents and emissions should be reported to the appropriate government body. Effective measures should be in place to disseminate information to the public about the toxicity and emissions of waterpipe tobacco smoking.

ADVISORY NOTE: Water tobacco smoking:
health effects, research needs and recommended actions for regulators

Article 11.1 a	**Health claims on packaging and labelling.** In accordance with Article 11 of the WHO FCTC, Parties should prohibit manufacturers and third parties from making health claims for waterpipe tobacco smoking and should prohibit deceptive descriptors that infer claims of health or safety (e.g. "contains 0% tar or 0.05% nicotine"). This must also apply to accessories, including claims made for charcoal ("odourless", "free of chemicals", "100% natural"). Even "tobacco free" or "herbal" waterpipe alternatives contain large doses of toxicants, and the packaging should not be allowed to carry health or safety claims.
b	**Health warnings on packaging and labelling.** Health warnings should indicate the various harmful effects of tobacco use and should: –be approved by a competent regulatory body; –be rotated at set intervals (e.g. every 12 months); –be large, clear, legible and visible; –cover no less than 30% of the principal display area (i.e. not hidden on the bottom or side where it might not be seen); and –be in the form of or including pictures or pictograms. Warning labels must be placed on waterpipe tobacco packaging and also on all accessories and on waterpipes themselves. Labelling waterpipe tobacco is not sufficient, as smokers may not see the packaging (if they smoke in a bar or café). As waterpipe parts, charcoal, filters and mouthpieces can be sold separately, warning labels should be affixed to all individual packaging. Regulation should go beyond the placement of warning labels on waterpipes. Waterpipes are considered aesthetically pleasing as well as functional, and manufacturers and smokers may resist or remove labelling that is considered to mar the beauty of the waterpipe. This should not be allowed. Because waterpipes present a novel challenge in terms of the placement of warning labels (on the waterpipe itself as well as accessories), pre-market testing of warning label placement would be useful, as would monitoring of placement options found to be successful in trials.
Article 12 a	Comprehensive education and public awareness programmes on the dangers of waterpipe smoking should be implemented. Programmes should specifically address the fallacy that waterpipe smoking is safer or healthier than smoking cigarettes.
b	Education and programmes for and about the benefits of cessation should be widely available.

c	Training on and awareness of the dangers of waterpipe smoking should be provided for health workers, community workers, social workers, media professionals, educators, decision-makers, administrators and all those who are pivotal in tobacco control and health care.
Article 13 a	Any form of waterpipe advertising, promotion and sponsorship must be regulated by an appropriate government body. This can be done most easily by making certain that waterpipes are included in all legislation and regulations governing cigarette advertising, promotion and sponsorship, without exception.
b	The regulations must be adapted to the unique feature of waterpipe vending, namely, that most advertising, promotion and sales are through the Internet.
c	At a minimum, Parties' regulations on advertising, promotion and sponsorship of waterpipes must: –not make them appealing to or target, either explicitly or implicitly, –non-smokers or non-nicotine users; –not make them appealing to or target, either explicitly or implicitly, minors, including through the selection of media, the location or the context in which they appear or through imagery that promotes sexual or sporting prowess; –encourage quitting smoking, and provide a quitline number if one exists; –not contain health, safety or medicinal claims; –not undermine any tobacco control measure, including not promoting exemption of waterpipe cafés from clean indoor air policies; –include factual information about the product's ingredients in a way that does not distort evidence of risks; –not link these products with gambling, alcohol, illicit drugs or activities or locations in which using them would be unsafe or unwise; –clearly state the addictive nature of nicotine and that these products are intended to deliver nicotine; and prohibit suggestions that waterpipes have positive qualities.
d	All authorized forms of waterpipe advertising, promotion and sponsorship must be cleared by the appropriate authority prior to publication or transmission in order proactively to prevent inappropriate marketing and then monitored to assess compliance with approval.
Article 14	Cessation programmes for tobacco dependence should include waterpipe tobacco smoking dependence. The interventions should target the unique features that make waterpipe smoking appealing and thus difficult to quit: –the appeal of the aroma, –the pleasant bubbling sound and –the social atmosphere or bonding and sharing over a waterpipe.

12. References

1. WHO Study Group on Tobacco Product Regulation (TobReg). Advisory note. Waterpipe tobacco smoking: health effects, research needs and recommended actions by regulators. Geneva: World Health Organization; 2005.

2. Control and prevention of waterpipe tobacco products (document FCTC/COP/6/11). Conference of the Parties to the WHO Framework Convention on Tobacco Control, Sixth session, Moscow, Russian Federation, 13–18 October 2014. Geneva: World Health Organization; 2014.

3. Goodman J. Tobacco in history: the cultures of dependence. London: Routledge; 1993.

4. Benedict CA. Golden-silk smoke: a history of tobacco in China. Berkeley, California: University of California Press; 2011.

5. Bhonsle RB, Murti PR, Gupta PC. Tobacco habits in India. In: Gupta PC, Hamner JE III, Murti PR, editors. Control of tobacco-related cancers and other diseases, proceedings of an international symposium. Bombay: Oxford University Press; 1992.

6. Chattopadhyay A. Emperor Akbar as a healer and his eminent physicians. Bull Indian Inst History Med 2000;30:151–8.

7. Maziak W, Eissenberg T, Ward KD. Patterns of waterpipe use and dependence: implications for intervention development. Pharmacol Biochem Behav 2005;80:173–9.

8. Rastam S, Ward KD, Eissenberg T, Maziak W. Estimating the beginning of the waterpipe epidemic in Syria. BMC Public Health 2004;4:32.

9. Maziak W, Taleb ZB, Bahelah R, Islam F, Jaber R, Auf R, et al. The global epidemiology of waterpipe smoking. Tob Control 2015;24(Suppl 1):i3–12.

10. Martinasek MP, McDermott RJ, Martini L. Waterpipe (hookah) tobacco smoking among youth. Curr Probl Pediatr Adolesc Health Care 2011;41:34–57.

11. Sutfin EL, Song EY, Reboussin BA, Wolfson M. What are young adults smoking in their hookahs? A latent class analysis of substances smoked. Addict Behav 2014;39:1191–6.

12. Akl E, Ward KD, Bteddini D, Khaliel R, Alexander AC, Loutfi T, et al. The allure of the waterpipe: a narrative review of factors affecting the epidemic rise in waterpipe smoking among young persons globally. Tob Control 2015;24(Suppl 1):i13–21.

13. Maziak W, Ward K, Soweid RAA, Eissenberg T. Tobacco smoking using a waterpipe: a reemerging strain in a global epidemic. Tob Control 2004;13:327–33.

14. Maziak W, Nakkash R, Bahelah R, Husseini A, Fanous N, Eissenberg T. Tobacco in the Arab world: old and new epidemics amidst policy paralysis. Health Policy Plan 2013;29:784–94.

15. Carroll MV, Chang J, Sidani JE, Barnett TE, Soule E, Balbach E, et al. Reigniting tobacco ritual: waterpipe tobacco smoking establishment culture in the United States. Nicotine Tob Res 2014;16:1549–58.

16. Afifi R, Khalil J, Fouad F, Hammal F, Jarallah Y, Abu Farhat H, et al. Social norms and attitudes linked to waterpipe use in the Eastern Mediterranean Region. Soc Sci Med 2013;98:125–34.

17. Tobacco policy trend alert. An emerging deadly trend: waterpipe tobacco use. Chicago, Illinois: American Lung Association; 2007 (http://www.lungusa2.org/embargo/slati/ Trendalert_Waterpipes.pdf, accessed 5 July 2014).

18. Nakkash RT, Khalil J, Afifi RA. The rise in narghile (shisha, hookah) waterpipe tobacco smoking: a qualitative study of perceptions of smokers and non smokers. BMC Public Health 2011;11:315.

19. Sutfin E, McCoy TP, Reboussin BA, Wagoner KG, Spangler J, Wolfson M. Prevalence and correlates of waterpipe tobacco smoking by college students in North Carolina. Drug Alcohol Depend 2011;115:131–6.

20. Salloum RG, Osman A, Maziak W, Thrasher JF. How popular is waterpipe tobacco smoking? Findings from Internet search queries. Tob Control. 2014 Jul 22. pii: tobaccocontrol-2014-051675. doi: 10.1136/tobaccocontrol-2014-051675.

21. Primack BA, Rice KR, Shensa A, Carroll MV, DePenna EJ, Nakkash R, et al. US hookah tobacco smoking establishments advertised on the Internet. Am J Prev Med 2012;42:150–6.

22. Carroll MV, Shensa A, Primack BA. A comparison of cigarette- and hookah-related videos on YouTube. Tob Control 2013;22:319–23.

23. Brockman LN, Pumper MA, Christakis DA, Moreno MA. Hookah's new popularity among US college students: a pilot study of the characteristics of hookah smokers and their Facebook displays. BMJ Open 2012;2. pii: e001709.

24. Salloum RG, Nakkash RT, Myers AE, Wood KA, Ribisl KM. Point-of-sale tobacco advertising in Beirut, Lebanon following a national advertising ban. BMC Public Health 2013;13:534.

25. Bahelah R. Waterpipe tobacco labeling and packaging and World Health Organization Framework Convention on Tobacco Control (WHO FCTC): a call for action. Addiction 2014;109:333.

26. Sepetdjian E, Shihadeh A, Saliba NA. Measurement of 16 polycyclic aromatic hydrocarbons in narghile waterpipe tobacco smoke. Food Chem Toxicol 2008;46:1582–90.

27. Knishkowy B, Amitai Y. Water-pipe (narghile) smoking: an emerging health risk behavior. Pediatrics 2005;116:e113–9.

28. Chaloupka FJ, Straif K, Leon ME. Effectiveness of tax and price policies in tobacco control. Tob Control 2011;20:235–8.

29. Gilmore AB, Tavakoly B, Taylor G, Reed H. Understanding tobacco industry pricing strategy and whether it undermines tobacco tax policy: the example of the UK cigarette market. Addiction 2013;108:1317–26.

30. El-Awa F, Warren C, Jones N. Changes in tobacco use among 13–15-year-olds between 1999 and 2007: findings from the Eastern Mediterranean Region. East Med

Health J 2010;16:266-73.

31. Akl EA, Gunukula SK, Aleem S, Obeid R, Abou Jaoude P, Honeine R, et al. The prevalence of waterpipe tobacco smoking among the general and specific populations: a systematic review. BMC Public Health 2011;11:244.

32. Maziak W. The waterpipe: time for action. Addiction 2008;103:1763-7.

33. Maziak W. The global epidemic of waterpipe smoking. Addict Behav 2011;36:1-5.

34. Morton J, Song Y, Fouad H, Awa FE, Abou El Naga R, et al. Cross country comparison of waterpipe use: nationally representative data from 13 low and middle-income countries from the Global Adult Tobacco Survey (GATS). Tob Control 2014;23:419-27.

35. Attitudes of Europeans towards tobacco. Special Eurobarometer 385. Brussels: European Commission; 2012 (http://ec.europa.eu/health/tobacco/docs/eurobaro_attitudes_towards_ tobacco_2012_en.pdf).

36. Smith-Simone S, Maziak W, Ward KD, Eissenberg T. Waterpipe tobacco smoking: knowledge, attitudes, beliefs, and behavior in two US samples. Nicotine Tob Res 2008;10:393-8.

37. Maziak W, Ward KD, Eissenberg T. Factors related to frequency of narghile (waterpipe) use: the first insights on tobacco dependence in narghile users. Drug Alcohol Depend 2004;76:101-6.

38. Warren CW, Lea V, Lee J, Jones NR, Asma S, McKenna M. Change in tobacco use among 13-15 year olds between 1999 and 2008: findings from the Global Youth Tobacco Survey. Global Health Promot 2009;16(Suppl):38-90.

39. Rice VH, Weglicki LS, Templin T, Hammad A, Jamil H, Kulwicki A. Predictors of Arab American adolescent tobacco use. Merrill-Palmer Q J Dev Psychol 2006;52:327-42.

40. Weglicki LS, Templin T, Hammad A, Jamil H, Abou-Mediene S, Farroukh M, et al. Tobacco use patterns among high school students: Do Arab American youth differ? Ethnicity Dis 2007; 17(Suppl 3): 22-4.

41. Rice VH, Templin T, Hammad A, Weglicki L, Jamil H, Abou-Mediene S. Collabo-

rative research of tobacco use and its predictors in Arab and non-Arab American 9th graders. Ethnicity Dis 2007;17(Suppl):19–21.

42. El-Roueiheb Z, Tamim H, Kanj M, Jabbour S, Alayan I, Musharrafieh U. Cigarette and waterpipe smoking among Lebanese adolescents, a crosssectional study, 2003–2004. Nicotine Tob Res 2008;10:309–14.

43. Primack BA, Sidani J, Agarwal AA, Shadel WG, Donny EC, Eissenberg TE. Prevalence of and associations with waterpipe tobacco smoking among US university students. Ann Behav Med 2008;36:81–6.

44. Zoughaib SS, Adib SM, Jabbour J. Prevalence and determinants of water pipe or narghile use among students in Beirut's southern suburbs. J Med Liban 2004;52:142–8.

45. Tamim H, Al-Sahab B, Akkary G, Ghanem M, Tamim N, El Roueiheb Z, et al. Cigarette and nargileh smoking practices among school students in Beirut, Lebanon. Am J Health Behav 2007;31:56–63.

46. Taha AZA. Prevalence of risk-taking behaviors. Bahrain Med Bull 2007;29:1–10.

47. Jackson D, Aveyard P. Waterpipe smoking in students: prevalence, risk factors, symptoms of addiction, and smoke intake. Evidence from one British university. BMC Public Health 2008;8:174.

48. Jawaid A, Zafar AM, Rehman TU, Nazir MR, Ghafoor ZA, Afzal O, et al. Knowledge, attitudes and practice of university students regarding waterpipe smoking in Pakistan. Int J Tuberc Lung Dis 2008;12:1077–84.

49. Senkubuge F, Ayo-Yusuf OA, Louwagie GM, Okuyemi KS. Water pipe and smokeless tobacco use among medical students in South Africa. Nicotine Tob Res 2012;14:755–760.

50. Combrink A, Irwin N, Laudin G, Naidoo K, Plagerson S, Mathee A. High prevalence of hookah smoking among secondary school students in a disadvantaged community in Johannesburg. S Afr Med J 2010;100:297–9.

51. Daniels K, Roman N. A descriptive study of the perceptions and behaviors of waterpipe use by university students in the Western Cape, South Africa. Tob In-

duced Dis 2013;11:4.

52. Global adult tobacco survey: Nigeria country report 2012. Brazzaville: World Health Organization Regional Office for Africa.

53. Khattab A, Javaid A, Iraqi G, Alzaabi A, Ben Kheder A, Koniski ML, et al. Smoking habits in the Middle East and North Africa: results of the BREATHE study. Respir Med 2012;106(Suppl 2):S16–24.

54. Czoli CD, Leatherdale ST, Rynard V. Bidi and hookah use among Canadian youth: findings from the 2010 Canadian Youth Smoking Survey. Prev Chronic Dis 2013;10:120290.

55. Agaku IT, King BA, Husten CG, Bunnell R, Ambrose BK, Hu SS, et al. Tobacco product use among adults—United States, 2012–2013. Morbid Mortal Wkly Rep 2014;63:542–7.

56. Amrock SM, Gordon T, Zelikoff JT, Weitzman M. Hookah use among adolescents in the United States: results of a national survey. Nicotine Tob Res 2014;16:231–7.

57. Palamar JJ, Zhou S, Sherman S, Weitzman M. Hookah use among US high school seniors. Pediatrics 2014;134:1–8.

58. Global Adult Tobacco Survey: Argentina 2012. Buenos Aires: Government of Argentina, 2013.

59. Shihadeh A, Azar S, Antonios C, Haddad A. Towards a topographical model of narghile water-pipe café smoking: a pilot study in a high socioeconomic status neighborhood of Beirut, Lebanon. Biochem Pharmacol Behav 2004;79:75–82.

60. Warren C, Jones N, Eriksen M, Asma S. Patterns of global tobacco use in young people and implications for future chronic disease burden in adults. Lancet 2006;367:749–53.

61. Mzayek F, Khader Y, Eissenberg T, Al Ali R, Ward KD, Maziak W. Patterns of water-pipe and cigarette smoking initiation in schoolchildren: Irbid Longitudinal Smoking Study. Nicotine Tob Res 2012;14:448–54.

62. Moh'd Al-Mulla A, Abdou Helmy S, Al-Lawati J, Al Nasser S, Ali Abdel Rahman S, Almutawa A, et al. Prevalence of tobacco use among students aged 13–15 years in

Health Ministers' Council/Gulf Cooperation Council Member States, 2001–2004. J School Health 2008;78:337–43.

63. Global Adult Tobacco Survey: Egypt country report 2009. Cairo: World Health Organization Regional Office for the Eastern Mediterranean.

64. Global Adult Tobacco Survey: GATS Qatar 2013 fact sheet. Doha: Government of Qatar.

65. Sorina I, editor. Global Adult Tobacco Survey—Romania 2011. Cluj-Napoca: Eikon, 2012.

66. Jawad M, Abass J, Hariri A, Rajasooriar KG, Salmasi H, Millett C, et al. Waterpipe smoking prevalence and attitudes amongst medical students in London. Int J Tuberc Lung Dis 2013;17:137–40.

67. Jawad M, Wilson A, Lee LT, Jawad S, Hamilton FL, Millet C. Prevalence and predictors of water pipe and cigarette smoking among secondary school students in London. Nicotine Tob Res 2013;15:2069–75.

68. Slama K, David-Tchouda S, Plassart J. Tobacco consumption among young adults in the two French departments of Savoie in 2008. Rev Epidémiol Santé Publique 2009;57:299–304.

69. Pärna K, Usin J, Ringmets I. Cigarette and waterpipe smoking among adolescents in Estonia: HBSC survey results, 1994–2006. BMC Public Health 2008;8:392.

70. Varsano S, Ganz I, Eldor N, Garenkin M. Water-pipe tobacco smoking among school children in Israel: frequencies, habits, and attitudes. Harefuah 2003;142:736–41.

71. Korn L. The nargila smoking phenomenon among teen-agers in Israel: a sociological analysis. PhD thesis. Ramat-Gan: Bar-Ilan University, Department of Sociology and Anthropology; 2005.

72. Korn L, Harel-Fisch Y, Amitai G. Social and behavioral determinants of nargila (water-pipe) smoking among Israeli youth: findings from the 2002 HBSC survey. J Subst Use 2008;13:225–38.

73. Harel Y, Molcho M, Tillinger E. Youth in Israel. Health, well-being and risk be-

haviors. Summary of findings from the third national study (2002) and trend analysis (1994–2002). Ramat-Gan: Bar-Ilan University, Department of Sociology and Anthropology; 2003.

74. Global Adult Tobacco Survey: Indonesia Report 2011. New Delhi: World Health Organization Regional Office for South East Asia.

75. GATS India Report 2009–2010. New Delhi: Ministry of Health and Family Welfare, Government of India; 2011.

76. She J, Yang P, Wang Y, Qin X, Fan J, Wang Y, et al. Chinese waterpipe smoking and the risk of chronic obstructive pulmonary disease. Chest 2014;146:924–31.

77. Report of the Global Adult Tobacco Survey (GATS) Malaysia, 2011. Kuala Lumpur: Institute for Public Health, Ministry of Health Malaysia; 2012.

78. Personal habits and indoor combustions. IARC Monographs on the Carcinogenic Risk of Chemicals to Humans, Vol. 100E. Lyon: International Agency for Research on Cancer; 2012.

79. Kassem NOF, Kassem NO, Jackson SR, Liles S, Daffa RM, Zarth AT, et al. Benzene uptake in hookah smokers and non-smokers attending hookah social events: regulatory implications. Cancer Epidemiol Biomarkers Prev 2014;146:924–31.

80. Saleh R, Shihadeh A. Elevated toxicant yields with narghile waterpipes smoked using a plastic hose. Food Chem Toxicol 2008;46:1461–6.

81. Apsley A, Galea KS, Sánchez Jiménez A, Semple S, Wareing H, Tongeren MV. Assessment of polycyclic aromatic hydrocarbons, carbon monoxide, nicotine, metal contents and particle size distribution of mainstream shisha smoke. J Environ Health Res 2011;11:93.

82. Jenkins R, Guerin M, Tomkins B. The chemistry of environmental tobacco smoke. Boca Raton, Florida: Lewis Publishers; 2000.

83. Monzer B, Sepetdjian E, Saliba N, Shihadeh A. Charcoal emissions as a source of CO and carcinogenic PAH in mainstream narghile waterpipe smoke. Food Chem Toxicol 2008; 46:2991–5.

84. Schubert J, Hahn J, Dettbarn G, Seidel A, Luch A, Schulz TG. Mainstream smoke

of the waterpipe: Does this environmental matrix reveal as significant source of toxic compounds? Toxicol Lett 2001;205:279–84.

85. Shihadeh A. Investigation of mainstream smoke aerosol of the argileh water pipe. Food Chem Toxicol 2003;41:143–52.

86. Bentur L, Hellou E, Goldbart A, Pillar G, Monovich E, Salameh M, et al. Laboratory and clinical acute effects of active and passive indoor group water-pipe (narghile) smoking. Chest 2014;145:803–9.

87. St Helen G, Benowitz NL, Dains KM, Havel C, Peng M, Jacob P 3rd. Nicotine and carcinogen exposure after water pipe smoking in hookah bars. Cancer Epidemiol Biomarkers Prev 2014;23:1055–66.

88. Cobb CO, Sahmarani K, Eissenberg T, Shihadeh A. Acute toxicant exposure and cardiac autonomic dysfunction from smoking a single narghile waterpipe with tobacco and with a "healthy" tobacco-free alternative. Toxicol Lett 2012;215:70–5.

89. Al Ali R, Rastam S, Ibrahim I, Bazzi A, Fayad S, Shihadeh AL, et al. A comparative study of systemic carcinogen exposure in waterpipe smokers, cigarette smokers and non-smokers. Tob Control 2015;24:125–7.

90. Jacob P, Raddaha AHA, Dempsey D, Havel C, Peng M, Yu L, et al. Nicotine, carbon monoxide, and carcinogen exposure after a single use of a water pipe. Cancer Epidemiol Biomarkers Prev 2011;20:2345–53.

91. Jacob P, Raddaha AHA, Dempsey D, Havel C, Peng M, Yu L, et al. Comparison of nicotine and carcinogen exposure with water pipe and cigarette smoking. Cancer Epidemiol Biomarkers Prev 2013;22:765–72.

92. El Zaatari ZM, Chami HA, Zaatari, GS. Health effects associated with waterpipe smoking. Tob Control 2015;24(Suppl 1):i31–43.

93. Lim BL, Lim GH, Seow E. Case of carbon monoxide poisoning after smoking shisha. Int J Emerg Med 2009;2:121–2.

94. La Fauci G, Weiser G, Steiner IP, Shavit I. Carbon monoxide poisoning in narghile (water pipe) tobacco smokers. Can J Emerg Med 2012;14:57–9.

95. Alomari MA, Khabour OF, Alzoubi KH, Shqair DM, Eissenberg T. Central and

peripheral cardiovascular changes immediately after waterpipe smoking. Inhal Toxicol 2014;26:579–87.

96. Hakim F, Hellou E, Goldbart A, Katz R, Bentur Y, Bentur L. The acute effects of water-pipe smoking on the cardiorespiratory system. Chest 2011;139:775–81.

97. Eissenberg T, Shihadeh A. Waterpipe tobacco and cigarette smoking: direct comparison of toxicant exposure. Am J Prev Med 2009;37:518–23.

98. Al-Kubati M, Al-Kubati AS, Al'Absi M, Fišer B. The short-term effect of water-pipe smoking on the baroreflex control of heart rate in normotensives. Autonomic Neurosci 2006;126:146–9.

99. Hawari FI, Obeidat NA, Ayub H, Ghonimat I, Eissenberg T, Dawahrah S, et al. The acute effects of waterpipe smoking on lung function and exercise capacity in a pilot study of healthy participants. Inhal Toxicol 2013;25:492–7.

100. Markowicz P, Löndahl J, Wierzbicka A, Suleiman R, Shihadeh A, Larsson L. A study on particles and some microbial markers in waterpipe tobacco smoke. Sci Total Environ 2014;499:107–13.

101. Fromme H, Dietrich S, Heitmann D, Dressel H, Diemer J, Schulz T, et al. Indoor air contamination during a waterpipe (narghile) smoking session. Food Chem Toxicol 2009;47:1636–41.

102. Cobb CO, Vansickel AR, Blank MD, Jentink K, Travers MJ, Eissenberg T. Indoor air quality in Virginia waterpipe cafes. Tob Control 2013;22:338–43.

103. Hammal F, Chappell A, Wild TC, Kindzierski W, Shihadeh A, Vanderhoek A, et al. "Herbal" but potentially hazardous: an analysis of the constituents and smoke emissions of tobaccofree waterpipe products and the air quality in the cafés where they are served. Tob Control 2015;24:290–7.

104. Maziak W, Ibrahim I, Rastam S, Ward KD, Eissenberg T. Waterpipe-associated particulate matter emissions. Nicotine Tob Res 2008;10:519–23.

105. Daher N, Saleh R, Jaroudi E, Sheheitli H, Badr T, Sepetdijan E, et al. Comparison of carcinogen, carbon monoxide, and ultrafine particle emissions from narghile waterpipe and cigarette smoking: sidestream smoke measurements and assess-

ADVISORY NOTE: Water tobacco smoking:
health effects, research needs and recommended actions for regulators

ment of second-hand smoke emission factors. Atmos Environ 2010;44:8–14.

106. Akl EA, Gaddam S, Gunukula SK, Honeine R, Jaoude PA, Irani J. The effects of waterpipe tobacco smoking on health outcomes: a systematic review. Int J Epidemiol 2010;39:834–57.

107. Dangi J, Kinnunen TH, Zavras AI. Challenges in global improvement of oral cancer outcomes: findings from rural northern India. Tob Induced Dis 2012;10:5.

108. Ali AA, Ali AA. Histopathologic changes in oral mucosa of Yemenis addicted to water-pipe and cigarette smoking in addition to takhzeen al-qat. Oral Surg Oral Med Oral Pathol Oral Radiol Endod 2007;103:e55–9.

109. Nasrollahzadeh D, Kamangar F, Aghcheli K, Sotoudeh M, Islami F, Abnet CC, et al. Opium, tobacco, and alcohol use in relation to oesophageal squamous cell carcinoma in a high-risk area of Iran. Br J Cancer 2008;98:1857–63.

110. Dar NA, Bhat GA, Shah IA, Iqbal B, Makhdoomi MA, Nisar I, et al. Hookah smoking, nass chewing, and oesophageal squamous cell carcinoma in Kashmir, India. Br J Cancer 2012;107:1618–23.

111. Malik MA, Upadhyay R, Mittal RD, Zargar SA, Mittal B. Association of xenobiotic metabolizing enzymes genetic polymorphisms with esophageal cancer in Kashmir Valley and influence of environmental factors. Nutr Cancer 2010;62:734–42.

112. Qiao YL, Taylor PR, Yao SX, Schatzkin A, Mao BL, Lubin J, et al. Relation of radon exposure and tobacco use to lung cancer among tin miners in Yunnan Province, China. Am J Ind Med 1989;16:511–21.

113. Gupta D, Boffetta P, Gaborieau V, Jindal SK. Risk factors of lung cancer in Chandigarh, India. Indian J Med Res 2001;113:142–50.

114. Lubin JH, Qiao YL, Taylor PR, Yao SX, Schatzkin A, Mao BL, et al. Quantitative evaluation of the radon and lung cancer association in a case control study of Chinese tin miners. Cancer Res 1990;50:174–80.

115. Lubin JH, Li JY, Xuan XZ, Cai SK, Luo QS, Yang LF, et al. Risk of lung cancer among cigarette and pipe smokers in southern China. Int J Cancer 1992;51:390–5.

116. Hsairi M, Achour N, Zouari B. Facteurs etiologiques du cancer bronchique prim-

itif en Tunisie. [Etiological factors for primary lung cancer in Tunisia.] Tunisie Med 1993;71:265–8.

117. Hazelton WD, Luebeck EG, Heidenreich WF, Moolgavkar SH. Analysis of a historical cohort of Chinese tin miners with arsenic, radon, cigarette smoke, and pipe smoke exposures using the biologically based two-stage clonal expansion model. Radiat Res 2001;156:78–94.

118. Sadjadi A, Derakhshan MH, Yazdanbod A, Boreiri M, Persaeian M, Babaei M, et al. Neglected role of hookah and opium in gastric carcinogenesis: a cohort study on risk factors and attributable fractions. Int J Cancer 2014;134:181–8.

119. Shakeri R, Malekzadeh R, Etemadi A, Nasrollahzadeh D, Aghcheli K, Sotoudeh M, et al. Opium: an emerging risk factor for gastric adenocarcinoma. Int J Cancer 2013;133:455–61.

120. Bedwani R, El-Khwsky F, Renganathan E, Braga C, Abu Seif HH, Abul Azm T, et al. Epidemiology of bladder cancer in Alexandria, Egypt: tobacco smoking. Int J Cancer 1997;73:64–7.

121. Zheng YL, Amr S, Saleh DA, Dash C, Ezzat S, Mikhail NN, et al. Urinary bladder cancer risk factors in Egypt: a multicenter case-control study. Cancer Epidemiol Biomarkers Prev 2012;21:537–46.

122. Mohammad Y, Shaaban R, Abou Al-Zahab B, Khaltaev N, Bousquet J, Dubaybo B. Impact of active and passive smoking as risk factors for asthma and COPD in women presenting to primary care in Syria: first report by the WHO-GARD survey group. Int J Chron Obstruct Pulmon Dis 2013;8: 473–82.

123. Waked M, Khayat G, Salameh P. Chronic obstructive pulmonary disease prevalence in Lebanon: a cross-sectional descriptive study. Clin Epidemiol 2011;3:315–23.

124. Tageldin MA, Nafti S, Khan JA, Nejjari C, Beji M, Mahboub B, et al. Distribution of COPDrelated symptoms in the Middle East and North Africa: results of the BREATHE study. Respir Med 2012;106(Suppl 2):S25–32.

125. Waked M, Salameh P, Aoun Z. Water-pipe (narguile) smokers in Lebanon: a pilot

study. East Med Health J 2009;15: 432–42.

126. Salameh P, Waked M, Khoury F, Akiki Z, Nasser Z, Abou Abass L, et al. Water-pipe smoking and dependence are associated with chronic bronchitis: a case–control study in Lebanon. East Med Health J 2012;18:996–1004.

127. Salameh P, Waked M, Khayat G, Dramaix M. Waterpipe smoking and depen-dence are associated with chronic obstructive pulmonary disease: a case–control study. Open Epidemiol J 2012;5:36–44.

128. Sekine Y, Katsura H, Koh E, Hiroshima K, Fujisawa T. Early detection of COPD is important for lung cancer surveillance. Eur Respir J 2012;39: 1230–40.

129. Sibai AM, Tohme RA, Almedawar MM, Itani T, Yassine SI, Nohra EA, et al. Lifetime cumulative exposure to waterpipe smoking is associated with coronary artery disease. Atherosclerosis 2014;234:454–60.

130. Wu F, Chen Y, Parvez F, Segers S, Argos M, Islam T, et al. A prospective study of tobacco smoking and mortality in Bangladesh. PLoS One 2013;8:e58516.

131. Islami F, Pourshams A, Vednathan R, Poustchi H, Kamangar F, Golozar A, et al. Smoking water-pipe, chewing nass and prevalence of heart disease: a cross-sec-tional analysis of baseline data from the Golestan Cohort Study, Iran. Heart 2013;99:272–8.

132. Selim GM, Fouad H, Ezzat S. Impact of shisha smoking on the extent of coronary artery disease in patients referred for coronary angiography. Anadolu Kardiyol Derg 2013;13:647–54.

133. El-Sadawy M, Ragab H, El-Toukhy H, El Latif El Mor A, Mangoud AM, Eissa MH, et al. Hepatitis C virus infection at Sharkia Governorate, Egypt: seropreva-lence and associated risk factors. J Egypt Soc Parasitol 2004;34(1 Suppl):367–84.

134. Habib M, Mohamed MK, Abdel-Aziz F, Magder LS, Abdel-Hamid M, Gamil F, et al. Hepatitis C virus infection in a community in the Nile Delta: risk factors for seropositivity. Hepatology 2001;33:248–53.

135. Medhat A, Shehata M, Magder LS, Mikhail N, Abdel-Baki M, Nafeh M, et al. Hepatitis C in a community in Upper Egypt: risk factors for infection. Am J Trop

Med Hyg 2002;66:633–8.

136. Steentoft J, Wittendorf J, Andersen JR. Tuberkulose og vandpibesmitte [Tuberculosis and water pipes as source of infection]. Ugeskr Laeg 2006;168:904–7.

137. Munckhof WJ, Konstaninos A, Wamsley M, Mortlock M, Gilpin C. A cluster of tuberculosis associated with use of a marijuana water pipe. Int J Tuberc Lung Dis 2003;7:860–5.

138. Salamé J, Salameh P, Khayat G, Waked M. Cigarette and waterpipe smoking decrease respiratory quality of life in adults: results from a national cross-sectional study. Pulm Med 2012;2012:868294.

139. Tavafian SS, Aghamolaei T, Zare S. Water pipe smoking and health-related quality of life: a population-based study. Arch Iran Med 2009;12:232–7.

140. Tamim H, Yunis KA, Chemaitelly H, Alameh M, Nassar AH, National Collaborative Perinatal Neonatal Network Beirut, Lebanon. Effect of narghile and cigarette smoking on newborn birthweight. B J Obst Gynaecol 2008;115:91–7.

141. Nuwayhid IA, Yamout B, Azar G, Kambris MA. Narghile (hubble-bubble) smoking, low birth weight, and other pregnancy outcomes. Am J Epidemiol 1998;148:375–83.

142. Aghamolaei T, Eftekhar H, Zare S. Risk factors associated with intrauterine growth retardation (IUGR) in Bandar Abbas. J Med Sci 2007;7:665–9.

143. Al-Belasy FA, Al-Belasy FA. The relationship of "shisha" (water pipe) smoking to postextraction dry socket. J Oral Maxillofac Surg 2004;62:10–4.

144. Natto S, Baljoon M, Bergstrom J. Tobacco smoking and periodontal bone height in a Saudi Arabian population. J Clin Periodontol 2005;32:1000–6.

145. Natto S, Baljoon M, Abanmy A, Bergstrom J. Tobacco smoking and gingival health in a Saudi Arabian population. Oral Health Prev Dent 2004;2:351–7.

146. Natto S, Baljoon M, Bergstrom J. Tobacco smoking and periodontal health in a Saudi Arabian population. J Periodontol 2005;76:1919–26.

147. Baljoon M, Natto S, Abanmy A, Bergström J. Smoking and vertical bone defects in a Saudi Arabian population. Oral Health Prev Dent 2005;3:173–82.

148. Tamim H, Musharrafieh U, El Roueiheb Z, Yunis K, Almawi WY. Exposure of children to environmental tobacco smoke (ETS) and its association with respiratory ailments. J Asthma 2003;40:571–6.

149. Islami F, Nasseri-Moghaddam S, Pourshams A, Poustchi H, Semnani S, et al. Determinants of gastroesophageal reflux disease, including hookah smoking and opium use—a cross-sectional analysis of 50,000 individuals. PLoS One 2014;9:e89256.

150. Primack BA, Land SR, Fan J, Kim KH, Rosen D. Associations of mental health problems with waterpipe tobacco and cigarette smoking among college students. Subst Use Misuse 2013;48:211–9.

151. Maziak W, Ward KD, Eissenberg T. Interventions for waterpipe smoking cessation. Cochrane Database Syst Rev 2011;6:CD005549.

152. Macaron C, Macaron Z, Maalouf MT, Macaron N, Moore A. Urinary cotinine in narguila or chicha tobacco smokers. J Med Liban 1997;45:19–20.

153. Maziak W, Rastam S, Shihadeh AL, Bazzi A, Ibrahim I, Zaatari GS, et al. Nicotine exposure in daily waterpipe smokers and its relation to puff topography. Addict Behav 2011;36:397–9.

154. Eissenberg T, Shihadeh A. Waterpipe tobacco and cigarette smoking: direct comparison of toxicant exposure. Am J Prev Med 2009;37:518–23.

155. Ward KD, Hammal F, VanderWeg MW, Eissenberg, Asfar T, Rastam S, et al. Are waterpipe users interested in quitting? Nicotine Tob Res 2005;7:149–56.

156. Maziak W, Rastam S, Ward KD, Shihadeh AL, Eissenberg T. CO exposure, puff topography, and subjective effects in waterpipe tobacco smokers. Nicotine Tob Res 2009;11:806–11.

157. Hammal F, Mock J, Ward KD, Eissenberg T, Maziak W. A pleasure among friends: how narghile (waterpipe) smoking differs from cigarette smoking in Syria. Tob Control 2008;17:e3.

158. Maynard OM, Gage SH, Munafò MR. Are waterpipe users tobacco-dependent? Addiction 2013;108:1886–7.

159. Maziak W, Ward KD, Afifi Soweid RA, Eissenberg T. Standardizing questionnaire items for the assessment of waterpipe tobacco use in epidemiological studies. Public Health 2005;119:400–4.

160. Salameh P, Waked M, Aoun Z. Waterpipe smoking: construction and validation of the Lebanon Waterpipe Dependence Scale (LWDS-11). Nicotine Tob Res 2008;10:149–58.

161. Primack BA, Khabour OF, Alzoubi KH, Switzer GE, Shensa A, Carroll MV, et al. The LWDS-10J: reliability and validity of the Lebanon Waterpipe Dependence Scale among university students in Jordan. Nicotine Tob Res 2014;16:915–22.

162. Aboaziza E, Eissenberg T. Waterpipe tobacco smoking: what is the evidence that it supports nicotine/tobacco dependence? Tob Control 2014;24(Suppl 1):i144–53.

163. Salameh P, Khayat G, Waked M. Lower prevalence of cigarette and waterpipe smoking, but a higher risk of waterpipe dependence in Lebanese adult women than in men. Women Health 2012;52:135–50.

164. Cobb C, Ward KD, Maziak W, Shihadeh AL, Eissenberg T. Waterpipe tobacco smoking: an emerging health crisis in the United States. Am J Health Behav 2010;34:275–85.

165. Asfar T, VanderWeg MW, Maziak W, Hammal F, Eissenberg T, Ward KD. Outcomes and adherence in Syria's first smoking cessation trial. Am J Health Behav 2008;32:146–56.

166. Rastam S, Eissenberg T, Ibrahim I, Ward KD, Khalil R, Maziak W. Comparative analysis of waterpipe and cigarette suppression of abstinence and craving symptoms. Addict Behav 2011;36:555–9.

167. Jaber R, Madhivanan P, Veledar E, Khader Y, Mzayek F, Maziak W. Waterpipe a gateway to cigarette smoking among adolescents in Irbid, Jordan: a longitudinal study. Int J Tuberc Lung Dis 2015;19:481–7.

168. Soneji S, Sargent JD, Tanski SE, Primack BA. Associations between initial water pipe tobacco smoking and snus use and subsequent cigarette smoking: results from a longitudinal study of US adolescents and young adults. JAMA Pediatr

2015;169:129–36.

169. Shihadeh AL, Eissenberg TE. Significance of smoking machine toxicant yields to blood-level exposure in water pipe tobacco smokers. Cancer Epidemiol Biomarkers Prev 2011;20:2457–60.

170. Zyoud SH, Al-Jabi SW, Sweileh WM. Bibliometric analysis of scientific publications on waterpipe (narghile, shisha, hookah) tobacco smoking during the period 2003–2012. Tob Induced Dis 2014;12:7.

171. Pepper JK, Eissenberg T. Waterpipes and electronic cigarettes: increasing prevalence and expanding science. Chem Res Toxicol 2014;27:1336–43.

172. Jawad M, McEwen MN, Shahab L. To what extent should waterpipe tobacco smoking become a public health priority? Addiction 2013;108:1873–84.

173. WHO Tobacco Laboratory Network. Standard operating procedure for determination of nicotine in cigarette tobacco filler. WHO Tobacco Laboratory Network (TobLabNet) official method. Standard operating procedure 04. Geneva: World Health Organization; 2014.

174. WHO Tobacco Laboratory Network. Standard operating procedure for determination of tobacco-specific nitrosamines in mainstream cigarette smoke under ISO and intense smoking conditions. WHO Tobacco Laboratory Network (TobLabNet) official method. Standard operating procedure 03. Geneva: World Health Organization; 2014.

175. WHO Tobacco Laboratory Network. Standard operating procedure for determination of benzo[a]pyrene in mainstream cigarette smoke under ISO and intense smoking conditions. WHO Tobacco Laboratory Network (TobLabNet) official method. Standard operating procedure 05. Geneva: World Health Organization; 2015.

176. Further development of the partial guidelines for implementation of Articles 9 and 10 of the WHO FCTC (Decision FCTC/COP6(12)). Conference of the Parties to the WHO Framework Convention on Tobacco Control, Sixth session, Moscow, Russian Federation, 13–18 October 2014. Geneva: World Health Orga-

nization; 2014.

177. Shihadeh A, Schubert J, Klaiany J, El Sabban M, Luch A, Saliba NA. Toxicant content, physical properties and biological activity of waterpipe tobacco smoke and its tobacco-free alternatives. Tob Control 2014;24:e72–80.

178. Khabour O, Alzoubi KH, Bani-Ahmad M, Dodin A, Eissenberg T, Shihadeh A. Acute exposure to waterpipe tobacco smoke induces changes in the oxidative and inflammatory markers in mouse lung. Inhal Toxicol 2012; 24:667–75.

179. Control and prevention of waterpipe tobacco products (Decision FCTC/COP6(10)). Conference of the Parties to the WHO Framework Convention on Tobacco Control, Sixth session, Moscow, Russian Federation, 13–18 October 2014. Geneva: World Health Organization; 2014.